From
LPN
to
RN

From
LPN
to
RN

Role Transitions

Kathy L. Ham, MSN, RN

Doctoral Candidate
University of Memphis
Memphis, Tennessee
Assistant Professor, Department of Nursing
Southeast Missouri State University
Cape Girardeau, Missouri

W.B. SAUNDERS COMPANY
A Harcourt Health Sciences Company

Philadelphia   London   New York   St. Louis   Sydney   Toronto

W.B. Saunders Company
A Harcourt Health Sciences Company

The Curtis Center
Independence Square West
Philadelphia, Pennsylvania 19106

Library of Congress Cataloging-in-Publication Data

Ham, Kathy.
  From LPN to RN : role transitions / Kathy Ham.
    p. ; cm.
  ISBN 0-7216-8739-3
    1. Nursing. 2. Nursing—Vocational guidance. 3. Career development. I. Title.
  [DNLM: 1. Nursing. 2. Career Mobility. 3. Nursing, Practical. WY 16 H198L 2002]
  RT82.H349 2002
  610.73—dc21

  2001032079

Vice President and Publishing Director, Nursing: Sally Schrefer
Senior Editor: Terri Wood
Developmental Editor: Frances Murphy
Illustrator: Keith Lesko

FROM LPN TO RN: ROLE TRANSITIONS   ISBN 0-7216-8739-3

Printed in the United States of America

Last digit is the print number: 9   8   7   6   5   4   3   2   1

To my husband, Cliff:

You not only encouraged me to do this, but also made it possible.

Thanks for being my biggest supporter,

Love, Kathy

Preface

For six years, I taught in an LPN to RN bridge program at Park University in Sikeston, Missouri. Each time I prepared to teach the introductory course of the one-year associate degree program, I was reminded of the scarcity of available materials that would address the specific needs of LPN/LVNs in a transition program to become RNs.

My colleagues and I used a variety of textbooks from which we obtained lecture material on such topics as nursing process, role transition, legal/ethical aspects of nursing, and adult teaching/learning principles. Unfortunately, it was neither cost-effective nor convenient for the students to purchase the large number of textbooks upon which we based our lectures. In addition, the texts appeared more suited to the traditional, generic registered nursing student.

It is my hope that this textbook will provide faculty and students the resource that has been needed to assist LPN/LVNs to successfully "bridge" to RN practice. The ten chapters contain material that may either be used to teach an introductory course on transition from LPN/LVN to RN, or be incorporated at later points within the program of study. In other words, chapters are free-standing and may be used in the order in which they work best for each nursing program's curriculum plan. It has been my desire to create a textbook that speaks directly to the LPN/LVN who is returning to school. The chapters on role transition, survival skills, and thinking skills have been written with such a person in mind.

The writing style speaks directly to the student in hopes of creating a sense of personal involvement in the educational process. Many LPN/LVNs enter a bridge program with some type of previous nursing experience; therefore, client scenarios and questions have been included within the chapters to stimulate thinking and allow for interactive learning. In chapter 1, students are introduced to three hypothetical students—Maria, Kevin, and Suzanna—who experience many of the same academic and personal concerns as real-life LPN to RN bridge students. Each successive chapter begins with dialogue among the three, who become a small support system for each other.

Despite the large number of men currently in nursing, I have often referred to the nurse as "she" unless otherwise designated. Thus I have tried to avoid the use of "he/she" each time a nurse is mentioned to streamline the reading.

In addition to the many opportunities for students to read questions and respond throughout the text, the end of each chapter contains critical thinking questions that encourage students to synthesize and respond to learned material in a written manner. The questions may be used as the starting point for classroom discussion, as many require an individualized answer based on previous personal nursing experiences. Answers to the critical thinking questions are provided in the accompanying instructor's manual. The instructor's manual, available free to faculty who adopt the text, also includes information on implementing the LPN/LVN to RN bridge program and a test bank of approximately 200 multiple-choice test questions.

I hope the material contained within this text provides helpful information for faculty who are teaching in LPN to RN transition programs, as well as the students who will be participating in the educational experience.

Kathy L. Ham, MSN, RN

Acknowledgments

Many people provided assistance and encouragement that have been invaluable to the completion of this work:

To the nursing students who ignited within me the desire to take on the task of writing a textbook, I thank you for giving me countless moments of personal satisfaction as a teacher. It has been wonderful to see you learn and grow as professionals.

To nursing colleagues, both past and present, I am grateful for your wisdom, guidance, and support. Special thanks go to Dr. Elaine Jackson, Dr. A. Louise Hart, and Dr. Janet Weber at Southeast Missouri State University for encouraging me to act on what was a rough beginning of a manuscript and for answering content questions.

To my editors at W.B. Saunders, Terri Wood, Fran Murphy, and Tom Stringer, you believed in me and were always available to offer suggestions and advice. Thank you for the opportunity to bring this idea to fruition. You made what seemed like an overwhelming task actually very accomplishable.

To the nursing staff at Missouri Delta Medical Center in Sikeston, Missouri, and Linda Boyd and her students of the practical nursing program of Sikeston Public Schools, many thanks for agreeing to assist with the photographs. You made wonderful models!

To Kathy Vickery, RN, MSN, goes a very special thank you for organizing the photography shoots and making that particular aspect of the project much easier.

And finally, I am especially indebted to my family for all the love and support I have received during my professional endeavors: My parents, Pete and Frances

Britt, always encouraged me to be independent and aim as high as I wanted; my mother-in-law, Peggy Ham, assisted with countless meals and babysitting; and my children, Jessica, Dale, and Jordan, gave me the opportunity to round out my life by being a mother. And one more time, thank you, Cliff.

KLH

Reviewers

Flora Adams, RNC
Skagit Valley College
Mount Vernon, Washington

Nancy J. Beverage, RN, MSN
De Anza College
Cupertino, California
El Camino Hospital
Cupertino, California

Donna Campbell, RN, MN
Columbia Basin College
Pasco, Washington

Nancy L. Cowan, RN, BSN, MSN, EdD
Chabot College
Hayward, California

Deborah Ford, RN, MS, MN, CCRN
Pasadena City College
Pasadena, California

Allen M. Hamilton, MS, BSN, RN
Distance Learning Instructor for McLennan Community College
Waco, Texas

Marjorie Knox, RN, MA, MPA
Community College of Rhode Island
Warwick, Rhode Island

Helen Kuebel, MSN, RN
Lower Columbia College
Longview, Washington

Mary Regina Jenette, RN, EdD, MA, MSN
West Virginia Northern Community College
Wheeling, West Virginia

Jo-Ann E. Landburg, MSN, MEd, RN, NCC
Western Nevada Community College
Carson City, Nevada

Gwen Lapham-Alcorn, RN, PhD
Central Florida Community College
Ocala, Florida

Fran Leibfreid, MEd, BSN, RN
Allegany College of Maryland
Cumberland, Maryland

Joan C. Oliver, EdD, RN
Mt. Hood Community College
Gresham, Oregon

Anne Ryan, MSN, RNC, MPH
Chesapeake College
Wye Mills, Maryland

Georgia Schilling, RN, BSN, MA
North Central Missouri College
Trenton, Missouri

Linda S. Smith, MSN, DSN, RN
Oregon Health Sciences University
Klamath Falls, Oregon

Sharon Souter, RN, MSN
New Mexico State University at
  Carlsbad
Carlsbad, New Mexico

Alice Stjernstrom, RN, MSN
Tyler Junior College
Tyler, Texas

Mildred R. Wade, MS, RN
Western Nevada Community
  College
Carson City, Nevada

Nancy A. Zavacki, RN, MSN
Central Oregon Community
  College
Bend, Oregon

Contents

From
LPN
to
RN

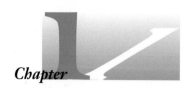

Chapter

Role Transition

LEARNING OBJECTIVES

After completing this chapter, you will be able to:

1. Discuss the concept of role transition from practical/vocational nurse to registered nurse.
2. Describe various role elements that are inherent in the scope of registered nursing practice.
3. Compare and contrast differences in role responsibilities of practical/vocational and registered nurses.
4. Describe the process of professional socialization from practical/vocational nurse to that of registered nurse.

Advocate	Educator	Role
Care Provider	Entrepreneur	Role Conflict
Change Agent	Manager	Role Model
Collaborator	Mentor	Role Transition
Counselor	Professional Socialization	
Critical Thinking	Researcher	

The decision to undertake a course of study that leads to a new role in nursing is not an easy one. It requires a tremendous commitment of time, energy, and financial resources, so you may need to put portions of your personal and professional life on hold. And you may feel uncertain about your ability to succeed.

Registered nurses wear a wide variety of "hats", and the nature of those hats is probably a little unclear to you at this time. But that will quickly change. You will be exposed to new responsibilities and new ways of thinking that will seem overwhelming at first. However, with practice and experience, you will suddenly find yourself viewing the world of nursing in a completely different way.

This chapter is intended to ease the role transition from licensed practical/vocational nurse (LPN/LVN) to registered nurse (RN). The road from LPN/LVN to RN is a difficult but manageable one. A journey of this kind requires an understanding of the major differences between the two roles, especially those related to the thinking processes inherent in each. Before beginning this trip, take time to open your mind to new ways of thinking and behaving. A closed mind will be your greatest obstacle. You have summoned the courage for this great undertaking. If you hang onto that courage as you encounter new territory, you will be successful.

ROLE SOCIALIZATION

Each of us functions in a variety of roles in life—mother, father, teacher, cub scout leader, and so on. A role carries a set of expectations that define the behavior society deems appropriate or inappropriate for the occupant. With each role comes a set of behaviors that help us formulate our performance to meet society's expectations. Nurses, both LPN/LVNs and RNs, also have roles. And the passage or transition from one nursing role to another involves a change in behavior—a change that must take place over a period of time in order for you, the student, to embrace the new role fully (Schumacher and Meleis, 1994).

As a child you may have seen pictures of capped nurses in starched white uniforms, or you may have watched television shows in which nurses were portrayed as hospital employees subservient to physicians. These images tend to influence our perceptions of what nursing is all about. Take a few moments to answer the following questions:

How have these early images influenced your expectations of yourself and other nurses?

_____

_____

_____

_____

_____

Did your practical/vocational nursing program support your preformed images about nursing, or did it challenge them? If so, how?

_____

_____

_____

_____

_____

As a practical/vocational nursing student, you acquired certain attributes that you judged to be important to a nurse. You may value characteristics such as a strong work ethic, ability to organize, efficiency, kindness, and dependability as necessary ingredients in the make-up of a good nurse. These are all desirable traits; but as a registered nurse, you'll be adding a broader range of qualities. In order to be successful as a registered nurse, you must be willing to build on attributes associated with your current understanding of nursing (Figure 1–1). For example, practical/vocational nursing education has provided you with the skills to observe for and report abnormalities in a client's vital signs. After transition to the registered nursing level, you will have developed problem solving skills that allow you to act on the information in a manner that will most benefit the client.

The transition from practical/vocational to registered nurse involves shaping, modifying, and adding information in order to achieve a more comprehensive view of client care. During this process, you will learn new ways of thinking while adapting to and accepting new behaviors within yourself. Take advantage

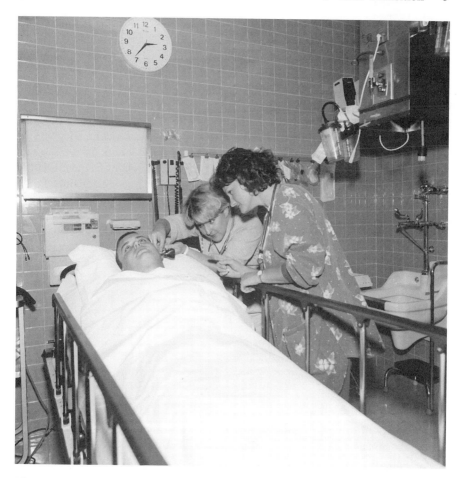

Figure 1-1
LPN to RN bridge students learn client assessment skills.

of the learning opportunities provided in your course of study and accept advice from your instructors, for they are your strongest allies at this time in your life. Feedback, positive or negative, is designed to help you move forward toward your goal of becoming a registered nurse.

Frequently, students encounter feelings of **role conflict,** especially when confronted with incompatible role requirements. Your friends, families, and co-workers have formed an image of you as a nurse on the basis of previous role behaviors. Upon entering a registered nursing program, you may unknowingly begin to change those behaviors as you learn to stretch your mind and assume new characteristics. You may be expected to perform in a new manner in your educational setting, even while those who know you best are still looking for the "old" you.

Therefore, the process of role transformation may be stressful when you encounter difficulties in meeting culturally defined role requirements. Uncorrected role strain can lead to chronic frustration and a sense of insecurity. As a student in role transition, consider finding ways to educate your family and friends about the changes that are occurring within you. Share your progress in learning new information and skills with your family. Usually, they will be eager to see the results of your labors, especially if those labors have taken you away from them for periods of time. And add to your circle of friends. Identify other students who are also in role transition and form a support group. You'll be surprised at the strong friendships that are forged from such relationships (Box 1–1).

As your journey leads you closer to becoming a registered nurse, you will gradually stop "role playing" as a student and the new role will becomes a part of you. That is, it will be internalized. And with internalization of the behaviors

Box 1-1   *Developing a Support Group*

 On the first day of classes of an LPN/LVN to RN bridge program at a local community college, three students discover they live within about one mile of each other in the same city. After brief introductions, they decide to meet at lunch and get better acquainted:

- Maria—a 40-year-old wife and mother of three teenagers—has worked 20 years as an LPN at a long-term care facility. She shares her dream of many years of becoming an RN, and expresses great fear at returning to school at her age.
- Kevin—a 32-year-old divorced father of a three-year-old daughter— says he plans to become a nurse practitioner eventually. He has four years' experience as an LPN and has been working twelve-hour weekend shifts in order to share custody of his daughter.
- Suzanna—a 19-year-old new graduate of a practical nursing program— has never had any client care experience other than nursing school. She is single, lives at home with her parents, and does not plan to work during the bridge program.

The three agree to carpool to classes and form a study group. Each states that s/he hopes to learn from the others' strengths as well as share his/her own. Please follow Maria, Kevin, and Suzanna through succeeding chapters as they experience the transition from practical to registered nurse.

and attitudes of a registered nurse comes the end of your journey along the path of role transition. But first, you have to begin the journey. And to do that, it will help to take a look at the role of registered nurse in its many aspects.

ROLE ELEMENTS

At this point, the concept of a role may seem a little abstract—you may even be wondering if you are going to be enlightened as to what exactly makes up a registered nurse. (You will.) Right now, however, let's begin with you. What do you think? Are registered nurses really so different from practical/vocational nurses? Please take a few minutes to answer the following question:

From your previous experiences, how do you view a registered nurse's duties and responsibilities as differing from those of a practical/vocational nurse?

_____

_____

_____

_____

_____

Actually, the role of registered nurse contains many parts, much like the many sparkling facets of a diamond. Each diamond facet lends its brilliant quality to that of the others to form one shining gem. Without each part, the diamond would not be as appealing. The many components that make up the role of the registered nurse combine to create the final product, a valuable member of the health care team (Figure 1–2).

Probably the most commonly recognized function of the nurse is that of **care provider.** Regardless of the setting, nurses are involved in a variety of activities that are aimed at one primary goal: ensuring the best possible health for the client. Care provider responsibilities in an out-patient clinic may include such functions as health screening, health promotion, and nursing interventions aimed at restoration of health. In the acute care setting, the registered nurse as a care provider must also be concerned with planning care for the entire family, such as on an obstetric unit. Traditionally, the care provider function of nursing—that of actually carrying out interventions that assist clients to meet positive outcomes—has been considered the essence of nursing.

By virtue of their frequent contact with clients and families, nurses are exposed to the personal joys and sorrows that occur during times of illness. Faced with navigating a confusing health care system, clients and families rely on nurses for guidance and support at such times. Therefore, the function of the registered

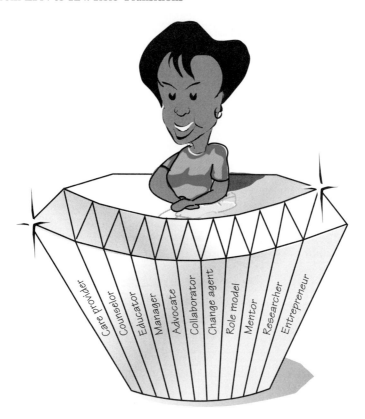

Figure 1-2
The multifaceted components of the role of registered nurse.

nurse as a counselor is a significant one. Registered nurses have an educational foundation of scientific knowledge that assists them in identifying clients' emotional needs. Therapeutic communication skills are a vital aspect of nursing care because many clients have psychosocial needs that are just as important as their physical needs (see chapter 5).

In today's rapidly changing world, clients must become more actively involved in their own health care than ever before. This means they need to be as informed as possible about aspects of care once thought to be beyond the comprehension of the general public. The nurse, then, is an educator, one who is in an excellent position to provide clients with much needed information about medications, dietary restrictions, treatments, and the like. Whether involved in formal client education classes, teaching community CPR courses, or answering a new mother's questions about breastfeeding, the registered nurse performs an essential educator function (see chapter 8 for more on client teaching).

Nurses make up the largest body of workers in today's health care facilities, and are generally looked to for leadership and organizational skills. The **manager** component of registered nursing involves not only supervising other members of the health care team, but also planning and coordinating care for groups of clients, families, and communities. Nurses guide and direct care at several levels, from team leader on a nursing unit to chief nursing officer in an acute care facility. In the community, registered nurses function as case managers and coordinators of groups of clients and staff. To be an effective manager, the nurse should possess sound decision making and problem solving skills, which are vital to optimal care planning. Chapter 9 provides a more detailed discussion of nursing leadership and management.

The registered nurse as an **advocate** is a protector who is willing to shield the client and family from harm. In assuming this duty, the nurse chooses to provide complete, honest information to those in her care, and to speak up against any harmful or unnecessary forces that might impede progress toward a healthy state. A client advocate agrees to "take the side" of the health care recipient, and "stand up for" the client's rights to autonomy and self-determination. The oncology nurse who asks for an increase in pain medication for a timid client is functioning as an advocate, as is the ICU nurse who questions a medical order to perform several procedures in one morning on a fatigued client.

As a valued member of the health care team, the registered nurse functions as a **collaborator** of care with physicians, assistive nursing personnel, pharmacists, physical therapists, social workers, and others. Collaboration involves working toward a common goal or end point, which is optimal health or compassionate end-of-life care for the client and family. Along with other colleagues, registered nurses participate in multidisciplinary meetings to set goals for clients to help achieve earlier discharge from the health care system. Finally, nurses collaborate with clients and families to plan care, in order to ensure cooperation and compliance.

Who is in a better position to sense needed change in a client care setting than the registered nurse? As a **change agent** (see chapter 9), the nurse must be willing to take risks when others are content with the status quo. Change is often resisted, and a nurse who has the energy, motivation, and interpersonal skills to persuade others to follow suit may not always be popular. However, health care organizations rely on their "frontline workers" to identify problems and make suggestions that could streamline work and contain costs. The registered nurse who possesses the courage to lead others in change is indeed a valuable asset to client care.

Another component of the registered nursing role is that of **role model**. When nurses present themselves to other nursing personnel in a manner that typifies the best attributes of the profession, they are said to be positive role models. Many characteristics have been suggested as desirable traits for registered nurses. For example, a nurse who upholds the American Nurses' Association (ANA) Code of Ethics (see chapter 10) and behaves in a caring, conscientious manner that always places the client first would be described as a good role model for others. It is particularly important that nursing students and new graduates into the profession be exposed to favorable role models.

A **mentor** is a trusted advisor (Zerwekh and Claborn, 1999). Especially when a nurse is being oriented to a new job, a mentor is important as someone who is available to counsel, teach, and promote professional growth. Generally, a mentor is a more experienced nurse who should be caring, nurturing, and concerned about the new nurse's development. An example of a mentor found in many health care organizations is a preceptor, who is usually responsible for new nursing employee orientation.

The **researcher** component of nursing involves investigating possible solutions to nursing and/or client problems. Most often, it is registered nurses who have obtained at least masters degree level education in nursing who engage in nursing research. However, it is the responsibility of all registered nurses to be aware of areas where research is needed in client care. For example, staff nurses on a medical unit should be willing to participate in clinical trials of new equipment, with the hope of improving care and reducing skyrocketing health care costs. Research helps us to find more efficient, effective ways to provide care, and helps us to better understand the nature of nursing.

Finally, a fairly new trend seen in nursing is that of the nurse **entrepreneur.** Many nurses have now formed their own businesses in home health, freestanding clinics, schools, and other areas. Nurse entrepreneurs function as con-

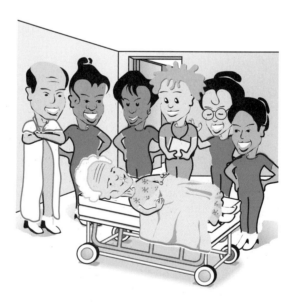

Figure 1–3
The nurse is a vital member of the health care team.

sultants, educators, and advisors to organizations and businesses who benefit from their services. This autonomous function of the registered nurse has provided more visibility for nursing to the general public and contributed to a more positive image.

Now, having learned a little about these eleven elements that make up the role of registered nurse, do you begin to see how your role as a practical/vocational nurse is about to expand? You may be thinking to yourself, "I do many of these things every day! Sure, maybe I don't get to be the charge nurse or do research, but who cares? I'm still a good nurse".

The issue here is not whether registered or practical/vocational nurses are more important, or who provides the better client care. As nurses, we are all valuable members of the health care team, and as such should focus on those aspects of nursing care that we are best equipped to provide (Figure 1–3). Registered nurses, by virtue of a more lengthy education, are taught to handle more complex client care problems, and have learned leadership skills necessary for guiding other nursing personnel through day-to-day concerns. In the next section, we'll look more closely at specific differences between the registered nurse and the practical/vocational nurse.

DIFFERENCES BETWEEN LPN/LVN AND RN ROLES

In the past, when asked to describe the differences in your duties as an LPN/LVN and those of RNs with whom you have worked, you may have been hard pressed to come up with many variations in the roles. For example, most LPN/LVNs will answer that the major areas in which RN duties differ from theirs is in supervision, legal responsibilities, and IV therapy. However, there are several areas in which these two types of nurses differ (Box 1–2).

Traditionally, practical/vocational nursing programs focus on teaching the "how to" of client care, while the emphasis in registered nursing education is on understanding "why" (Hill and Howlett, 2001). Registered nurses are taught

Box 1-2 *Areas of Differences in LPN and RN Roles*

- Educational preparation
- Thinking skills
- Assessment skills
- Nursing care planning
- Legal responsibilities
- IV therapy
- Communication skills
- Client teaching skills

to use a variety of thinking skills to understand client problems and to plan and evaluate care. Whether a registered nursing program prepares a nurse at the associate, baccalaureate, masters, or doctoral degree level, it generally contains the following components that differ from a practical/vocational nursing program of study:

- College-level science courses that lay the groundwork for an understanding of psychosocial and physiological aspects of client care.
- College-level liberal arts and general education courses to improve communication skills and encourage a holistic approach to client care.
- Nursing courses designed to provide an understanding of complex disease processes and client needs.
- Additional clinical hours in which to practice the role of registered nurse under the guidance of an instructor.

Registered nurses are educated to function in a variety of settings, such as clients' homes, hospitals, clinics, and long-term care facilities. They have been taught to handle complex client problems that require a broad scope of knowledge. Even though practical/vocational nurses are primarily prepared to practice nursing in a more structured environment under the direction of an RN, they frequently care for clients in the same settings as RNs.

A second difference between RNs and LPN/LVNs is in the orientation to use of thinking skills. Registered nursing programs accredited by the National League for Nursing are required to provide evidence that **critical thinking** is being taught throughout their curricula. The term "critical thinking" is widely used and broadly interpreted in all aspects of education in the United States. You may be asking yourself, "What exactly is critical thinking?" and "How do I learn to do it?"

Richard Paul (1992), a leading author in the field of critical thinking, defines it as "the art of thinking about your thinking while you are thinking in order to make your thinking better". In other words, critical thinking involves more than simply making routine decisions or judgments. It requires that the nurse be able to evaluate each element of the thinking process to ensure high standards of thinking. In addition, critical thinking involves rationally analyzing information before reaching a conclusion. Please read the following client scenario and answer the questions:

> Nellie Austin, an 86-year-old client on a skilled nursing unit, has been repeatedly calling for pain medications since her admission to the unit one day earlier. Tom Carey, the nurse on the evening shift, checks her record and finds that she is five days post-op from repair of a fractured hip. He notices that she has been receiving oral narcotics for pain management, and that her last dose was administered three hours previously. The physician's order reads to administer the medication every four hours as needed for pain.

Discuss what you would do if you were Ms. Austin's nurse in this situation, giving a rationale for your action(s):

_____

_____

_____

_____

_____

List the steps involved in your thinking process:

_____

_____

_____

_____

_____

Was it difficult for you to analyze the steps involved in your thinking process? Most of us are not taught to analyze and reflect upon how we think. Several choices are possible for this scenario. Tom could have:

- Followed the physician's order and withheld medication for one more hour.
- Asked another nurse for advice.
- Called the physician to request additional pain medication.
- Gathered more information in order to choose the best course of action.

Critical thinking calls for gathering all the facts related to the situation and the use of rational judgment to make a decision. Registered nurses must rely on critical thinking skills on a daily basis in order to provide optimal client care (Alfaro-LeFevre, 1999). Because practical/vocational nursing programs are shorter than registered nursing programs, less time is available for discussions of critical thinking and for practice in making sound judgments based on facts.

Actually, there are several kinds of thinking skills that should be incorporated into a nursing program of study in order for the graduate to be best prepared to deal with today's challenging world of health care. Chapter 6 discusses critical thinking; it also describes the need for nurses to possess creative thinking as well as problem solving and decision making skills. The registered nurse, as a team leader, is responsible for utilizing clear, analytical thinking abilities to guide others in planning client care.

Assessment skills, the third area of differences between LPN/LVNs and RNs, also vary with the amount of education and clinical practice time. For legal purposes, registered nurses must complete and sign the nursing assessment portion of a client's chart. In many instances, however, practical/vocational nurses perform a basic nursing assessment, including vital signs. Once again you may be wondering how your nursing assessment as an LPN/LVN could be different from that of an RN when you complete the same paperwork on clients. Perhaps this story from a student in an LPN to RN bridge program will assist you to understand:

> While I was studying to become an RN, I continued my job as an LPN at the hospital in my hometown. After about two months of returning to share what I was learning, I noticed that a good friend, who was also an LPN, began to avoid me. Finally, I stopped her in the hallway one day and asked why she never talked to me at work anymore. She replied, "You act like you know more than me now. I don't see how you can, when you're still doing the same things for clients that you did before you started back to school".
>
> After considering her comments for a short time, I explained, "Well, you know, I never knew I was acting differently, but I'm glad that I am, because I'm actually learning to be a different nurse than before. For example, when you listen to a client's breath sounds, what do you hear?" My friend replied, "I count the respiratory rate and make sure I hear sounds on both sides of the chest". To this I responded, "I do that too, but now I also know to make sure the breath sounds are equal, and to listen for such things as crackles, wheezes, and rubs. Because I'm learning more about disease processes, I can now relate more of what I'm hearing with what is wrong with my clients".

The registered nurse, with additional theory in pathophysiology and physical assessment, is better equipped than the practical/vocational nurse to evaluate a client's health status. Because of this knowledge base, she gathers a wide variety of information during an assessment of the client and family. Taking into account all aspects of a client's situation, from cultural and social factors to actual physical symptoms, the registered nurse utilizes a holistic approach to plan nursing care.

A fourth area of differences between RNs and LPN/LVNs is in nursing care planning. Practical/vocational nurses identify common client problems and participate in assisting clients to achieve expected outcomes in the plan of care. But registered nurses utilize problem solving skills to formulate a care plan, establish mutual goals with the client and family, and oversee the implementation and evaluation of the plan. Nursing diagnosis formulation is widely taught in registered nursing programs; but if introduced in practical/vocational nursing curricula, it is generally addressed in less depth. The RN, therefore, is more oriented toward leading other nursing personnel in designing, implementing, and evaluating the nursing plan of care.

Legally speaking, there are vast differences in RN and LPN/LVN functions. Even though LPN/LVNs are sometimes found in charge nurse positions in areas that utilize few RNs (such as long-term care facilities), they typically receive little preparation in management theory. Furthermore, state nurse practice acts do not generally recognize management as a common responsibility of the practical/vocational nurse. Team leader, charge nurse, nurse manager, and nurse administrator duties are usually assigned to registered nurses, who possess the required education and experience to make the decisions inherent in such positions. The final responsibility for client care rests with the nurse who functions in a role of authority in any given health care setting. Generally speaking, situations that require a higher level of nursing judgment are assigned to the RN.

Administration of intravenous (IV) therapy is another area of differing responsibilities among practical/vocational and registered nurses. Even though many states have allowed LPN/LVNs to administer IV medications after completing a course in IV therapy, legal considerations continue to suggest that RNs be involved in overseeing the administration of blood and various other IV medications. Registered nursing program curricula typically address IV therapy content in greater depth than do practical/vocational nursing programs. A greater understanding of drug interactions and complications of intravenous infusions better equips the RN to care for clients with IV therapy.

Another major area of differences in preparation of LPN/LVNs and RNs is in that of communication skills. Therapeutic communication theory is introduced at the LPN/LVN level in order to prepare students for interacting with clients and families. However, there is limited time to expand upon other aspects of communication that are important to client care (see chapter 5). Registered nurses, on the other hand, are exposed to theory on various normal and abnormal communication patterns, as well as mental health disorders. They also have the opportunity to care for clients experiencing behavioral difficulties while in mental health clinical rotations and, therefore, to practice communication skills. The RN completes courses in psychology and sociology in order to form a better understanding of behavioral cues that might influence communication. Therefore, the RN and LPN/LVN have been prepared differently to deal with the communication aspects of the nurse-client relationship.

Client teaching is an important function of nursing, but LPN/LVNs typically have not received theory regarding teaching-learning principles, or been taught to develop educationally oriented mutual goals with clients. Registered nurses are educated to observe for blocks to client readiness to learning, and to prepare an individualized teaching plan for the client that is realistic and achievable (chapter 8). RNs educate community groups on wellness topics, provide in-service classes to other health care personnel, and design nursing curricula for future members of the profession. LPN/LVNs are frequently given the responsibility of providing clients with information about diet, medications, and other aspects of self-care, but may not have been introduced to principles that enhance learning.

Are you beginning to realize that there are, in fact, many differences in what LPN/LVNs and RNs actually do? You, as an LPN/LVN, may be participating in nursing care planning and in giving clients discharge instructions for home care, but have you received the education needed to really understand what you are doing? Typically, LPN/LVNs who become students in an RN completion program relate that they quickly learn how inadequate their knowledge level was for some of the duties they have been asked to perform. As one student stated:

> I've eaten my words many times over for saying that I, as an LPN, did the same things as the RN I work with. I'm certified in IV therapy, but it's kind of scary now to see how much I didn't know about the IV medications I've been giving. After my instructor started requiring me to use a medication book to look up the administration rate of IV push medications before giving them, I realized I didn't have all the answers after all!

Each nurse makes important contributions to client care, regardless of the type of licensure. It is, however, important for you as a practical/vocational nurse who is moving into a registered nurse role to be able to see the differences between the two, and to be willing to learn new ways of thinking about nursing care. By developing an attitude of eagerness and willingness to assume new responsibilities, you may begin to truly see the benefits of reaching for a higher education.

PROFESSIONAL SOCIALIZATION

Now that you have examined the differences between LPN/LVN and RN roles, let's consider the **professional socialization** process you must undergo to become a registered nurse. *Formal socialization* into registered nursing, according to Chitty (1997), involves planned educational experiences, such as performing physical assessment, developing nursing diagnoses for a client's care plan, and doing client teaching. *Informal socialization*, on the other hand, includes lessons learned incidentally while you are functioning in a student role. You might, for example, learn to evaluate lab findings before administering medications by watching a staff nurse who has incorporated this practice into her routine. Or you might develop a better understanding of unprofessional behavior by overhearing staff nurses gossip about co-workers. In order for you to progress toward becoming a registered nurse, both types of socialization are necessary. To effectively embrace the role of registered nurse, you must take full advantage of both formal and informal socialization opportunities.

As a registered nursing student, you will begin to perform the routines and specific behaviors of the role. In order to do this, you must start to separate your thinking processes from those of task-oriented nursing, and move toward decision making and problem oriented client care. You will need to visualize yourself as a nurse who is capable of taking client care as far as possible in nursing, and no longer limit yourself to providing basic care and referring problems to an RN. In other words, your socialization into registered nursing will include formal lessons, informal types of learning, and a change in the way you view yourself.

Your pathway to professional socialization will take you through a process of movement through four stages before role transition occurs (Figure 1–4). As a student in a bridge program for practical/vocational nurses, you can expect to experience each stage to some extent. Depending on your personality and beliefs about nursing education, you may move through some stages faster than others.

Stage one begins when a practical/vocational nurse enters an LPN/LVN to RN completion program, or perhaps from the moment consideration is given to making application to the program. At this point, a variety of emotions are experienced, ranging from the excitement of a new challenge to the fear of failure. Along with the anxiety associated with a task of this nature, many students also begin the program with a certain amount of skepticism as to whether there really is much more to learn about being a nurse. Some have practiced for years, and are very confident about their abilities as nurses. Frequently, the more seasoned LPN/LVNs enter the program with a "show me" attitude, challenging the idea that there is truly more to be learned about nursing.

Early in an LPN/LVN to RN completion program, students usually begin to experience feelings of dissonance related to their abilities as nurses. Students enter stage two as more difficult material is presented, requiring them to look at nursing and nursing education in a manner with which they are unfamiliar. For example, many practical/vocational nurses in an RN program find they are not capable of achieving grades that are as high as those they received in their practical/vocational nursing program. As a result, they may feel they cannot succeed at that level, and become very anxious and frustrated. During clinical rotations many of the students tend to want to provide LPN/LVN level care to clients, and feel inadequate when challenged to analyze laboratory findings and explain disease processes in more depth than previously. Self-doubt and insecurity are typical emotions at this point in the process of professional socialization.

Stage three begins with a "letting go" of the practical/vocational nurse way of thinking and a dawning acceptance of thinking patterns and behaviors of the registered nurse. This requires that students develop self-insight into personal learning needs, and display a willingness to adopt new nursing knowledge and skills. As this acceptance of a new role takes place, students may begin to enjoy learning new information. Frequently, students become less frustrated and less anxious about their abilities to achieve their goal at this point, and appear to be more relaxed about the program of learning.

Finally, stage four occurs when the student completely adopts the attitudes and behaviors of the registered nurse. As a student, the practical/vocational nurse will be continuing to practice previous nursing behaviors and ways of thinking, but at this point, registered nursing characteristics will be incorporated into her everyday nursing practice. Many students actually say that they believe every nurse should be an RN, since they have found more pleasure in a higher

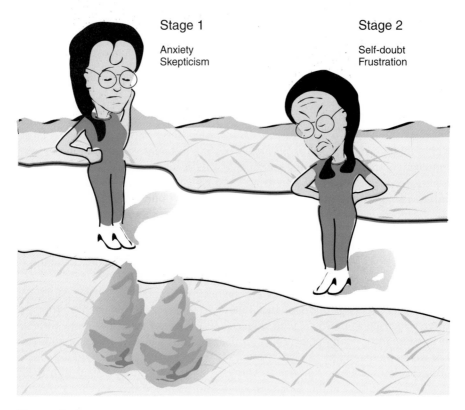

Figure 1–4
Stages of LPN/LVN to RN role transition.

level of nursing knowledge and feel more prepared to provide comprehensive care to clients.

The process of professional socialization from practical/vocational to registered nursing ends when you, the student, complete the four stages and enter a new role as a nurse. While moving along the road to this final goal, you will experience many emotions, which may be eased somewhat by remembering that a transition must occur during the process. Please allow yourself to participate fully in new experiences and take advantage of assistance from family, friends, fellow students, and nursing instructors. The world of nursing is opening up for you in ways you could not know before. Prepare yourself for new ways of planning, implementing, and evaluating client care as you assume the role of registered nurse. And good luck!

Stage 3

Self insight
Relaxation

Stage 4

Pleasure in learning
Self-assurance

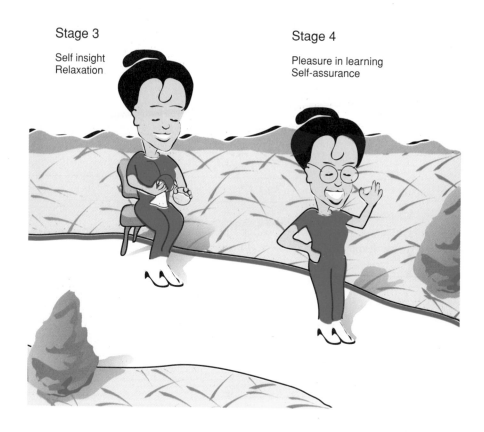

CRITICAL THINKING EXERCISES

1. Make a list of what you consider to be your LPN/LVN role attributes. How do you think these will change as you move toward becoming an RN?

_____

_____

_____

_____

_____

_____

2. Choose an RN with whom you have worked as an LPN/LVN and compare and contrast each of your responsibilities in client care. Underline RN role responsibilities that you believe will be the most difficult to learn.

_____

_____

_____

_____

_____

_____

3. Have you experienced any other times in your life when you had a role change? Explain. Describe the emotions you felt during the process.

_____

_____

_____

_____

_____

_____

4. Which people in your life will be your best support systems during this process? Why? Who will be least supportive? Why? How can you best use this information to ease your role transition from LPN/LVN to RN?

_____

_____

_____

_____

_____

_____

REFERENCES

Alfaro-LeFevre, R. (1999). *Critical thinking in nursing: A practical approach* (2nd ed.). Philadelphia: W.B. Saunders.

Chitty, K. (2001). *Professional nursing: Concepts and challenges* (3rd ed.). Philadelphia: W.B. Saunders.

Hill, S., and H. Howlett (2001). *Success in practical nursing: Personal and vocational issues* (4th ed.). Philadelphia: W.B. Saunders.

Paul, R. (1992). *Critical thinking: What every person needs to survive in a rapidly changing world* (2nd ed.). Santa Rosa, CA: Foundation for Critical Thinking.

Schumacher, K., and A. Meleis (1994). Transitions: A central concept in nursing. *Image* 26(2):119–127.

Zerwekh, J., and J. Claborn (1999). *Nursing today: Transition and trends* (3rd ed.). Philadelphia: W.B. Saunders.

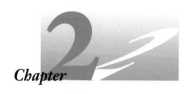

Chapter 2

Survival Skills for the Nontraditional Student

LEARNING OBJECTIVES

After completing this chapter, you will be able to:

1. Describe how the returning nontraditional college student differs from the traditional college student.
2. Discuss intrapersonal/interpersonal stressors that affect nontraditional college students.
3. Identify available resources to assist with the transition from practical/vocational nurse to registered nursing student in a college setting.
4. Discuss self-care measures designed to ease college life for the returning nursing student.
5. Explain the importance of developing effective study habits to success as a nursing student.

Academic Shock	Intrapersonal Stressors	Time Management
Distress	Nontraditional Student	Traditional Student
Eustress	Stress	
Interpersonal Stressors	Survival Skills	

 Maria, Kevin, and Suzanna are in a student lounge at college, awaiting their next class. They are attempting to find a common time that would be convenient for all to meet and study together.

Suzanna: What about Tuesday evening?

Maria: No, I have a Girl Scout meeting with my 13-year-old daughter on Tuesday nights. I'm a troop leader, so I have to be there.

Kevin: Well, we could meet at my apartment on Thursdays around 7 PM. What about then? My daughter stays with her mother that evening, so that's good for me.

Suzanna: My boyfriend and I go to the movies on Thursdays. That's his only evening free from work, so I can't just give that up. But the thing is, I'm really worried about my time! How do I get all my school work done every day and still have a normal life?

As the three friends continue to discuss a mutually satisfactory meeting time, it becomes obvious that each has personal commitments that must be considered when planning study sessions. Like most returning nontraditional students, they are faced with personal and professional obligations that can compete with academic demands, contributing to the stress of school.

Here you are—an LPN/LVN who has decided to further your education in order to become an RN. What factors prompted your decision? Was it the lure of higher pay? How about more professional recognition? Or maybe the decision was made for you by your employing agency.

Whatever the reason(s), if you've completed a practical/vocational nursing program, chances are it was in a vocational school or other higher education center, not a college setting. You may or may not have had the typical college experience . . . struggling through lengthy registration activities or sitting in a large lecture hall, lost among a hundred classmates. Returning to school to become a registered nurse may be a stressful experience in many ways.

As a practical/vocational nursing student, you may have had all your classes in one classroom, with no more than three or four instructors during the entire program. Your classes were designed to meet the needs of **nontraditional students,** or those who are older, self-sufficient in some way, and have more life experiences than typical college students. Most college classes are not specifically tailored to the needs of more mature learners; and if this is your first experience in such a setting, you may feel confused and isolated (Warner and Dishner, 1997). Add to this confusion the stress you will probably be experiencing as a result of role transition, and you may find yourself questioning your decision to begin this undertaking!

The purpose of this chapter is to examine specific needs of the nontraditional returning college student, and to provide helpful hints for being successful in such a program of study. Effective study habits, time management, and self-care strategies will be explored, specific to the needs of the practical/vocational nurse in a registered nursing program.

THE NONTRADITIONAL STUDENT IN COLLEGE

Returning to school is a major decision, as it will clearly bring about a change in everyday lifestyle. If you have an established routine that includes a job and/or family, this change can be unnerving. The social environment of a college is quite different from that of the work world, and you may experience feelings of isolation and insecurity.

If you are just being introduced to life at a college, you may find the process of acquiring an education to be as challenging outside the classroom as in. Making application for admission, registering for classes, and obtaining a parking permit are processes that can be time-consuming and frustrating. Nontraditional returning students often find that college offices are primarily open for business during the hours they work at jobs, and have difficulty obtaining textbooks and meeting with advisors (Snyder, 1992). Daily life can become a balancing act if you must plan childcare and a work schedule around college classes. In addition, the social mix of college students in non-nursing courses may cause you to feel out of place.

When you began your first job as a practical/vocational nurse, you may have experienced similar confusion; however, over time you have undoubtedly become more comfortable with your role. Now, as a returning student, you must begin to learn to interact in a new environment. This change frequently brings with it role confusion, anxiety, and feelings of self-doubt (de Wit, 1995).

One of the most frequent concerns expressed by practical/vocational nurses who are enrolled in an LPN to RN bridge program is self-doubt:

> I felt like I was a really good nurse until I started this program. Now I doubt my nursing abilities and feel dumb. I'm having trouble passing nursing exams. How can that be when I made good grades in LPN school?

A registered nursing program contains more rigorous course work, and students must usually carry several classes at the same time. The nontraditional student may find that younger, more **traditional students** seem to be at ease with such a schedule. Such students appear to have many advantages: They often live on campus, attend classes during the day, and do not work. This disparity can be overwhelming to the LPN/LVN who chooses to continue to work while attending school. In addition, the LPN/LVN to RN student may find that the practical/vocational nursing approach to client care is not always congruent with priorities presented in the classroom or clinical setting of the registered nursing program (de Wit, 1999). If you are an experienced practical/vocational nurse, you may find it difficult to change thinking patterns that you have used for many years.

Nontraditional students bring more life experiences to college than do their younger counterparts; therefore, they bring different needs to an academic program of study (Table 2–1). Often, they express resentment at being required to take courses that are not reality-based, since they need to be able to apply content directly to everyday life (Snyder, 1992). Traditional students, on the other hand, seem to be more tolerant of general studies courses that do not have immediate application to their chosen major.

As an LPN/LVN, you already have a major area of interest, and may fail to see the relevance of such courses as chemistry and English composition. If you take non-nursing courses with students from other majors, you may find your perspective on the content to be very different from theirs. Although these disparate viewpoints may be quite disconcerting at first, the encounter with different approaches actually encourages you to learn from others. As nurses,

TABLE 2-1
Differences in Nontraditional and Traditional Learners

NONTRADITIONAL	TRADITIONAL
Need a flexible course schedule	Flexibility in scheduling not as critical
Prefer reality-based course content and application of life experiences	Do not have as many life experiences to apply to learning opportunities
Require extended hours for accessing college support services	Utilize college support services primarily during work-day hours
Expect to actively participate in own education	Are usually passive rather than active learners

we tend to retreat into our own comfort zones when in a college setting, seeking out the company of other nurses. This comfort-seeking can help reduce the stress of returning to school; however, it can also limit your ability to broaden your horizons, which is what education is all about.

Nontraditional students also need help in creating links with the campus community (Warner and Dishner, 1997). They need to be able to feel a part of the college. A frequently voiced concern from returning nontraditional students is the lack of resources specific to their needs. Nontraditional students may not be very interested in new freshman orientation meetings, but they are often eager to obtain information on evening campus services. A course that is scheduled for one evening a week for three hours may be more manageable than one offered three times a week for one hour each day.

Many registered nursing programs are designed with courses in blocks, so working students do not have to attend classes five days a week. Evening and weekend programs offer another option for practical/vocational nurses who normally work Monday through Friday. Few nurses are willing to give up job seniority or comfortable hours if they continue to work while in school.

Based on comments from nontraditional learners, it would seem that they prefer to take an active part in their own education. Becoming part of a college's social and intellectual life involves a different process for nontraditional returning students than for traditional students, and brings concerns of a different nature.

THE STRESS OF RETURNING TO SCHOOL

As a practical/vocational nurse, you have experienced the day-to-day stress associated with nursing. High-acuity clients, inadequate staffing, and bureaucratic constraints are commonplace in today's health care arena. You have undoubtedly learned to handle these stressors based on your own individual coping skills. Returning to school at this point in your life will require a great deal of emotional and physical strength and determination. This is a task that can be accomplished, however, if you are able to identify and successfully manage stress.

Hans Selye described **stress** as "the non-specific response of the body to any demand made upon it" (Selye, 1976). This definition suggests that stress may be either good or bad. That is, it can hamper your ability to function effectively, or it may actually improve performance. **Eustress** is the term used to describe good, or positive, stress. For example, you experience eustress when you graduate from nursing school (doesn't that sound good?) or get a raise at work.

Nursing school can bring about a certain amount of positive stress. You may, for example, be feeling a new pride and an increased sense of self-worth because you have made the decision to further your education. Unfortunately, a certain amount of negative stress—**distress**—is also attached to the venture. Usually, individuals find ways to cope with negative stress; however, if distress is experienced for a prolonged period of time, personal relationships and health may suffer harmful effects.

Several factors are responsible for stress in the practical/vocational nurse enrolled in a registered nursing program. These factors can be grouped into the following categories: (1) personal stressors, (2) time management, (3) financial concerns, and (4) academic performance. Moreover, as shown in Figure 2–1, these categories are interrelated. For example, poor time management affects academic success, which can have an impact on personal relationships, and so

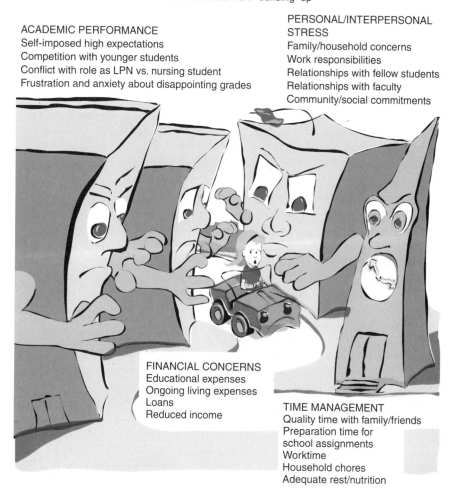

Prevent stress from "building" up

ACADEMIC PERFORMANCE
Self-imposed high expectations
Competition with younger students
Conflict with role as LPN vs. nursing student
Frustration and anxiety about disappointing grades

PERSONAL/INTERPERSONAL STRESS
Family/household concerns
Work responsibilities
Relationships with fellow students
Relationships with faculty
Community/social commitments

FINANCIAL CONCERNS
Educational expenses
Ongoing living expenses
Loans
Reduced income

TIME MANAGEMENT
Quality time with family/friends
Preparation time for school assignments
Worktime
Household chores
Adequate rest/nutrition

Figure 2–1
Areas of student stress.

forth. Students experience difficulties in each area to varying degrees, but many identify common problems. As you progress through nursing school, keep alert to the influences these stressors have on your life.

Personal Stressors

Returning to school may generate increased feelings of personal stress, which may manifest as either intrapersonal or interpersonal stress. The concerns you impose upon *yourself* are considered **intrapersonal stressors.** You may, for instance, be worrying about not making all A's or feel unsure about whether you can "cut it" as an RN. You may attend the first day of classes, receive course syllabi, listen to instructors' expectations, then go home and cry. If this happens, take comfort in the fact that this is common among nontraditional returning students. A major undertaking such as nursing school always seems overwhelming at first glance. An experienced LPN shared the following thoughts about her first day in an LPN to RN bridge nursing program:

> I had rearranged my entire life to go back to school, but after the first day I was afraid that I had made a big mistake. After worrying all evening, I decided the rest of my classmates didn't look any more capable than I did, so thought I would try a second day. Thankfully, I stuck it out and was able to finally graduate and become an RN, which was a long-time dream of mine.

Interpersonal stressors occur as a result of your interactions with others. Tension may develop between you and a best friend when you are forced to reduce social activities because of academic demands. Co-workers frequently view returning to school as a personal choice that should not interfere with commitments at work and do not understand when you must decline to work overtime. Other LPN/LVNs may express negativity toward you if they feel threatened by your new knowledge and skills. In addition, it may be confusing for you to function as an RN student a few days a week, only to return to work the following day as an LPN!

Another area of concern for the nontraditional student is that of abandoning family commitments. Married students experience stress because they miss children's extracurricular activities, evenings out with their spouses, and other quality family time. Time spent preparing nourishing meals at home may be replaced by picking up fast food. New babysitting arrangements may cause additional stress, especially when children are resistant to change. A demanding educational program can put a strain on a marriage, particularly if the student's spouse is not understanding and supportive of the endeavor.

Time Management

Time management is the second area of stress in nontraditional students. Many students continue to work, and find it difficult to squeeze everything that needs to be done into one day. What if you have to choose between completing a care plan assignment or going to work? Which will you sacrifice? If your five-year-old daughter has an asthma attack, will you be able to take an exam after spending the night in the Emergency Department? Nursing students are especially guilty of trying to take on too many responsibilities at once. As a result, they do not get enough rest, and place themselves at risk for poor health. The student who "burns the candle at both ends" does not perform well in any area of life.

Financial Concerns

Was the availability of financial support a determinant in your decision to further your education? How to pay for school while maintaining a reasonable lifestyle is a great concern for returning nontraditional students. Most college students currently receive some sort of financial assistance, in the form of loans or scholarships. Even if you have carefully calculated how much is needed for your education, you are likely to incur unexpected expenses. It is sometimes difficult, for example, to factor in the cost of gas or of meals eaten away from home. In addition, total family income may be reduced as a result of fewer hours worked on the job while in school.

Financial worries are a part of everyday life; however, the extra burden of tuition, books, and incidentals is especially taxing to the nontraditional student. Loan checks may arrive at later dates than expected, causing added pressure to meet financial obligations. Finally, life has a way of intruding into the best laid plans. Just when money is the tightest, your car breaks down on the way to school, gas prices double, and your student loan request is rejected.

Academic Performance

Anxieties produced by personal stresses, time management, or financial problems are usually intermittent, however acute. Stress over academic performance, however, seems to be continuous. Although students do report worrying about relationships, time, and money, their academic concerns are constant. One student related the following regarding coursework:

> It feels like I always have schoolwork hanging over me that is left undone. No matter how hard I try, I can't ever seem to get away from it. There is a constant feeling of pressure to get good grades. I guess that comes from within myself, since I want very much to do well in this program. Now that I'm older, I care more about grades than I used to. I know that I can make A's in my classes if I just work hard enough, but I never imagined there would be this much difference between LPN and RN classes. This is so much harder!

As indicated previously, a registered nursing program involves higher level material that requires a large time commitment. Most practical/vocational nurses are amazed at the volume and level of difficulty of the material required. For a number of students, having to write a formal paper is a frightening experience. Many expect to make the same grades as in their practical/vocational nursing program, only to be surprised when they receive their first exam scores. Practical/vocational nurses have reported feeling like "impostors" in a registered nursing program. The following student comment is an example:

> When we began to discuss the nursing process, I thought this would be easy, since I already use it at work. Imagine my surprise when I found out I had to develop nursing diagnoses with three-part statements! Even though we were studying pathophysiology, this was extremely hard for me. I felt that I had no right trying to be an RN, since I didn't think I would ever master the knowledge.

The stress experienced due to academic shock—feeling overwhelmed by the amount and difficulty level of schoolwork—can express itself in many forms. Students may become openly aggressive toward instructors, challenging them at every turn. They may also adopt passive-aggressive behaviors or direct their aggression internally. The passive-aggressive student displays aggressive behavior covertly, often turning in assignments late or chronically complaining. The internally aggressive student, however, may experience depression, feelings of hopelessness, and neglect proper self-care habits. It is not unusual to see these behaviors in a class of returning nursing students. Small groups of students tend to band together to gripe about assignments, argue over test questions, and in general to "buck the system." Others gain or lose weight or experience health problems.

When chronic maladaptive responses to stress continue over time, students may actually begin to feel themselves trapped in a situation over which they have little control. Needless energy is consumed in negative behaviors, and the ability to think and work effectively is altered. At a time when an astute mind and energetic body are most needed, students may feel as if their lives are spinning out of control.

SURVIVAL SKILLS

All human beings perceive a sense of comfort if they experience *homeostasis*—equilibrium, or a balance of elements—in their lives. In a student who has been exposed to chronic feelings of depression, hopelessness, or anger, the ability to self-regulate homeostasis may be absent or diminished.

Despite the upheaval a return to school can bring to your life, there are some simple strategies to help you hold it together. We will next examine survival skills that have proved helpful to the returning student who is a practical/vocational nurse. These tips, which have been contributed by former nursing students, address three areas: (1) getting organized, (2) taking care of yourself, and (3) adapting to the role of student (see Figure 2–2).

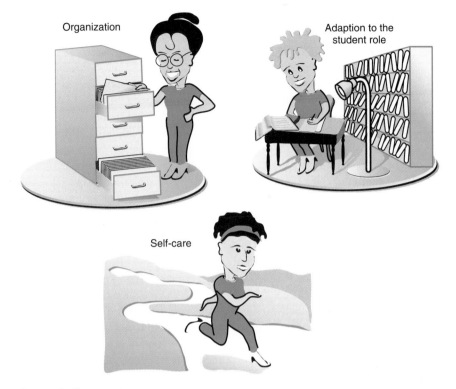

Organization

Adaption to the student role

Self-care

Figure 2–2
Three areas of survival skills.

Organization

Time management can be very challenging when the number of commitments increases dramatically in a brief period of time—a phenomenon that occurs when a working adult begins nursing school. The following list of suggestions is aimed at guiding you in getting organized so you can increase your productivity and reduce stress:

1. Buy a personal planner. It doesn't matter if you choose a month-at-a-glance, week-at-a-glance, or a daily calendar; just use whatever works best for you. Some students like to see the entire month, so they can write in major assignments, tests, and so forth. Others prefer to look at one week at a time so they do not feel so overwhelmed by what needs to be done. Regardless of your preference, you need to take each course syllabus and fill in all exams and assignment due dates to help you remember them.

You should also schedule periods each day for studying, exercise, and downtime with family/friends.

2. Use your calendar each day to identify and prioritize activities. Try to accomplish each without procrastination or wasted time. Sometimes it is helpful to promise yourself a treat if you complete everything as planned for the day. You might, for example, allow yourself to watch a favorite TV program as a reward for finishing all scheduled items.

3. Set up and use a separate work area at home for studying. Prior to the first day of classes, stock this area with all the supplies you need—pens, pencils, paper, a computer, and so forth—so you won't need to waste time shopping once the semester begins. Make sure there's space to store all your course materials in an organized fashion. For example, some students find it helpful to compartmentalize each course into separate boxes or folders (Zerwekh and Claborn, 1999). You also need room to spread out in. If you need to leave books open or half-finished papers out, you'll want to be assured your things won't be disturbed. Post messages of encouragement to yourself around your personal space: "The sooner I do it, the better I'll feel," "Take one bite at a time, and soon the meal will be finished," "Self-pity is self-destructive," "Motivation gets you started, habit keeps you going." Try purchasing a pair of earplugs to use during study time, especially if you live in an active household.

4. Whether you live alone or with others, prepare meals in advance. Try to find favorite recipes that can be frozen ahead of time. For example, while you are studying on Sunday afternoon, try preparing two or three stews, soups, or casseroles. Enlist the aid of others in preparation of meals. If you have children, this might be a good time to teach your children cooking skills!

5. Divide household chores with friends/family members with whom you live. If you're used to doing all the housework, try relaxing your standards: Learn to live with a dirty house, or delegate tasks to others. Even children as young as five or six can be taught to dust, empty the trash, and clear the dinner table. Work out any necessary babysitting arrangements in advance, and make sure you have backup help in case of emergency, especially if you are a single parent.

6. Before classes start, have your automobile serviced, tires checked, and make sure your insurance, license plate, and driver's license are current. Once school starts, you do not want to deal with car problems that could cost you money and lost class time. Whenever possible, carpool to and from classes, as this will save money and provide you with someone with whom to share school experiences.

7. Make sure you have a current CPR card, LPN/LVN license, health and malpractice insurance, completed immunizations, a checkup by a physician or nurse practitioner, and any other required documents prior to beginning

classes. These are necessary items in order to attend clinical experiences as a nursing student, and any delay on your part in producing them can jeopardize your ability to complete course requirements. The longer you wait to take care of turning these in, the more stress you bring upon yourself.

8. Do not use your only day off to catch up on all your errands, cooking, cleaning, and so forth. Do a few of these things each day so you'll have time to spend with others, take a nap, and recharge yourself (Figure 2–3).

9. Learn to say NO. At this time in your life, you do not need to be supernurse at work or to accept extra social responsibilities. Explain to friends and acquaintances that you need to put some activities on hold for the length of your nursing program. Tell yourself daily that you do not have to be perfect—it's okay to be adequate.

Self-Care

As you organize your daily activities to meet the demands of student life and its attendant changes, make sure you include healthy behaviors as a part of your routine. Perhaps it would be helpful to look at personal health from a holistic perspective, one that includes physical, mental, and spiritual components. The

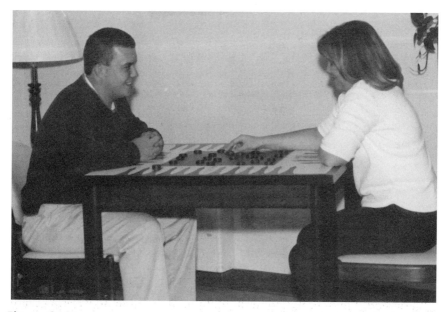

Figure 2-3
Leisure time helps maintain health.

following recommendations address areas of your life that should not be neglected, especially during a time of higher than normal stress:

1. Eat balanced meals as often as possible. It's easy to grab junk food when you're hurrying to class; however, it doesn't take that much time to tuck healthy foods—apples, cheese and crackers, yogurt—into your backpack. You might want to invest in a small lunch bag, one that holds a cold pack for perishables. If you pack your lunch bag ahead of time, it's very easy to slip it in your backpack as you leave for school. Try to include healthy drinks, such as fruit juices, as well. Avoid the urge to buy potato chips and sweets from vending machines during class breaks. Limit the number of caffeinated drinks you consume, as caffeine may increase stress.

2. Include time for daily exercise on your calendar. Taking a walk with a family member or friend is a good way to relax and refocus after a hectic day. Many colleges have gym facilities that are available for student use during free time. Whether or not you are already an exercise enthusiast, look for opportunities during the day for 20 to 30 minutes of activity that will benefit your body and relieve stress.

3. Get enough sleep each night. The rule of thumb for sleep is seven to eight hours per night, depending on your personal energy level. This means you should strive for at least this much in order to function well. Look for times during the day when you can rest and recharge; for example, try closing your eyes for 15 to 20 minutes in a quiet room. If you find it difficult to get as much sleep as you need, examine your daily activities: You may be procrastinating, putting off tasks until they intrude on your sleep time.

4. Set aside time each day to socialize with family and friends. This might include watching 30 minutes of cartoons with your child, going for a drive with your spouse, or visiting by phone with a faraway friend. It's amazing how much better you'll feel, both physically and mentally, simply by getting your mind off schoolwork for a period of time. Try to incorporate physical exercise into this time to receive additional benefits.

5. Do not neglect your spiritual self. Find the time to worship or meditate in the manner that best accommodates your lifestyle and personal beliefs. A sense of spiritual well-being will allow you to feel more positive about life and to look forward to the future (Zerwekh and Claborn, 1999).

6. Maintain good physical health by making regular appointments with your doctor/nurse practitioner and dentist for health screening exams. Attempt to keep your weight stable with exercise and proper nutrition. Limit alcohol intake and do not smoke if at all possible. Many students develop harmful habits, such as consuming more alcohol, caffeine, and nicotine due to the stress of school. In the long run, the effects of such behavior are not worth the temporary gratification experienced at the time of consumption.

7. Acknowledge the sources of stress in your life and take steps to keep them in check. Address issues that arise by using a problem solving approach to achieve resolution (see chapter 6). For example, a conflict with an instructor over a written assignment can be handled by taking specific steps: (a) identifying the problem, (b) gathering pertinent information, (c) meeting with the instructor to present the concern, (d) attempting to reach a mutually satisfying resolution, and (e) evaluating the outcome of the meeting and considering implications for future problems.

8. Face one day at a time instead of worrying about the entire week. Set priorities and ask for help when you need it. This is sometimes hard for nurses, who feel they must take care of everything alone.

9. Be your own personal cheerleader. Practice self-affirming statements daily (de Wit, 1999), such as: "I am important and special," "I am capable of changing and growing into a new person," and "I am free to develop to my greatest potential." Avoid negative influences at this time in your life, such as nonsupportive friends and co-workers.

10. Do not forget to build on your own strengths. You have experiences to share, and should not be afraid to do so (Bradshaw and Nugent, 1997). Do not be intimidated by what you consider to be self-weaknesses. Take an active part in your educational experience in order to get the most out of it.

11. Find the time to laugh. Listen to humorous radio programs while in your car, read a joke book during class breaks, or participate in a funny activity with friends. Consider this example:

> Following a classroom exam over particularly difficult material, eight nursing students gathered in the student parking lot, packed themselves into a small car, and tuned the radio to loud music. They rocked the car back and forth in beat with the music until they were laughing uproariously. In just five minutes, they had greatly reduced their stress levels. Returning to class shortly afterwards, they reported feeling more relaxed than previously. Perhaps there is truth to the saying "laughter is the best medicine."

Student Role

The final set of survival skills applies to your performance in the role of student. You have already reached the point where you are willing to make school a priority, and now you wish to perform to the best of your ability. Students who get the most from their educational experience are those who follow these suggestions:

1. Form collegial relationships with your instructors. They are available to guide and support you during the program of study (Copp, 1995). Take advantage of their expertise and advice. When you have questions or

concerns in a particular course, meet with that instructor immediately. During the meeting, present your concern maturely and professionally. Attacking, belligerent behavior is an improper way to communicate when trying to resolve a problem.

2. Treat instructors and fellow students with respect. Make appointments with instructors, rather than walking in unannounced. Be considerate of opinions expressed by your classmates. Do not participate in classroom gossip or other behaviors that contribute to a negative learning atmosphere.

3. Develop a support group of fellow students (see Box 1–1), preferably those who avoid maladaptive behaviors, such as constant griping and self-pity. School is stressful enough without exposing yourself to people who create more turmoil. Some students enjoy studying with a group; others do not. Your classmates can often help you understand a difficult concept about which you are unclear.

4. Participate in class. Ask questions when you do not understand something. Instructors may not be able to determine from your expression that you are confused, so speak up. Do the assigned readings before going to class, so you will be better prepared to discuss information as it is being presented.

5. Seek out new learning experiences. You may, for example, have helped with a lumbar puncture as an LPN/LVN; but if the opportunity arises to participate as an RN student, take advantage of it. Remember, you should start examining the world of nursing from a different perspective, so try viewing the lumbar puncture as an RN student. You should be beginning to have a greater understanding of the need for the procedure, the body's physiological response to the illness, and the nursing care involved.

6. Follow the school's dress code policy, as it has been developed to create professionally attired representatives of the nursing program. Becoming a registered nurse involves dressing and acting the part.

7. Take responsibility for your own learning. Do not expect to be spoonfed by your instructors. Accept criticism constructively and try to learn from it. Remember: *Trying* to do good work does not always guarantee that it *is* good work.

8. Familiarize yourself with available resources, such as the library, computer center, financial aid office, counseling and health centers, student center, and bookstore. Take advantage of these services in order to make college life easier.

Going back to school brings about many changes in your life, some easier to adjust to than others. Many of the frustrations encountered by you, the returning student, can be avoided by anticipating difficulties and being proactive, rather than reactive. The survival skills described here have been reported to be helpful by previous LPN to RN program students.

MANAGING THE ACADEMIC WORKLOAD

Most people have no formal training in how to study effectively and take tests; students learn these skills by trial and error. Despite a genuine desire to learn, students all too often invest large amounts of time engaging in ineffective studying. To their amazement, several hours' worth of test preparation does not necessarily guarantee a high grade.

If you are one of the many students who stay up most of the night before a test, trying to learn as much as possible at the last minute, you are studying incorrectly. You are not only exhausted, you are also failing to learn the material: You are merely attempting to memorize it, remembering it just long enough to do well on the test. Or perhaps you begin to research and write a formal paper two days before it is due. If so, do not plan on turning in your best work.

Academic work will take up a large part of your daily schedule as a nursing student. Be sure you plan carefully when filling in your calendar, allotting plenty of time for the number of hours needed to study and prepare for class.

Writing, studying, and test-taking are academic skills—skills that students can refine in order to perform better in school (Table 2–2). By using these three skills efficiently, students exercise their ability to assume control of their own work and take responsibility for their own learning (Nugent and Vitale, 1997). If you have a sense of being "in command" of the educational process, you have a great way to reduce the stress of school.

TABLE 2–2
Academic Skills

Writing Skills	• Case study papers
	• Term papers
	• Clinical logs
	• Nursing care plans
	• Journal article critiques
Studying	• Reading textbook assignments
	• Reviewing class notes
	• Reading related journal articles
	• Viewing audio-visual learning material
	• Participating in study groups
	• Working with tutors
	• Practicing nursing skills
Test-Taking	• Written in-class exams
	• Take-home exams
	• Nursing skills performance exams
	• Licensing/certification exams

Writing

As a college student you will be expected to write in a scholarly manner. If several years have passed since you wrote high school English papers, you might need to purchase a book on composition and grammar. Most returning nursing students suggest taking any required college English courses before the nursing component of the degree program. This will prepare you for writing nursing papers and free you from the extra burden of composing English papers while writing client care plans.

Does writing a formal written paper seem like busy work to you? Nursing faculty typically assign formal written papers for several reasons. First, you refine your research skills as you gather information for the paper. Second, preparing a paper gives you an opportunity to take an in-depth look at a particular aspect of nursing, whether it is a professional issue, disease process, or case study. Third, writing clarifies your thinking. Regardless of the focus of the assignment, learning occurs. In addition, written papers allow students more opportunity to show the instructor how much they know in a way that's less threatening than taking an in-class exam. Finally, students are generally afforded the chance to be somewhat creative in expressing themselves on written work, and that stimulates critical thinking.

When writing a formal paper, think of the assignment as a way to develop a product of which you want to be proud. If you consider the task a tedious, boring one, it will be. Try to approach the project with a sense of interest and inquiry. Box 2–1 contains suggestions to aid you in formal paper writing.

Studying

One of the major contributors to poor grades is insufficient, ineffective study time. You may feel that you already devote an extraordinary amount of time to

Box 2-1   *Guidelines for Writing Papers*

- Follow the instructions for the paper carefully and completely
- Start the assignment early; do not procrastinate
- Meet with the instructor to ask questions about the assignment, if needed
- Use a good typewriter or word processing computer program to type the paper
- Follow correct format as indicated by the instructor (many require APA, or American Psychological Association, format)
- Be as neat and legible as possible; correct all mistakes
- Use proper grammar and sentence structure; if unsure, get help
- Turn in the paper on time
- Meet with the instructor for questions about the grade

studying. But ask yourself: Are you spending that time well? In order for you to achieve the greatest benefit, you must learn how to utilize your time efficiently.

How do you prepare for class? Do you do assigned readings, view videos, practice case studies, and answer the questions located in your textbook? These are excellent ways to learn the material. The course syllabus should contain learning objectives and content material pertaining to each class session, together with assigned readings. It is very important that you make the time to complete these readings prior to coming to class.

Many times students complain that they find the readings overwhelming, both in quantity and complexity. Try keeping a medical dictionary handy for new or unfamiliar words. Stop and look up their definitions, and take the time to understand them. The following steps outline a useful method for reading material that is new:

1. Glance over the material first, reading headings, captions under photos, charts, diagrams, etc., to get an idea of the content to be read.
2. Read each section slowly, pausing at the end of each to consider major points, review definitions, and relate the concepts presented.
3. As you read, make a note of any unclear points. Take the notes with you to class so you may ask questions as the material is discussed.
4. Take time to read and think about any case studies and client care plans that are included with the material. Answer critical thinking exercises and practice exam questions, if provided.
5. Using the course syllabus, review objectives pertaining to the assignment you read. Make sure you can meet these objectives, as these should be the basis for course exams.
6. Do not panic if you do not have a good understanding of the assigned content at this time. Learning activities in class should help explain and reinforce the material you have read.
7. Just before class, glance back over content headings and words in bold to refresh your memory. As material is presented and discussed, ask questions about any unclear items.

As you take notes in class, do it in an organized fashion so you can read and understand them later. If you make a habit of reading assignments prior to class, note-taking is generally easier, because you already have some understanding of the material and you have some sense of its logical organization. You do not always need to write down every word said by the instructor in order to take good notes. Instead, listen attentively, and try to jot down major points. You can always go back to your textbook later to fill in gaps in your notes. Get together with a classmate to compare notes if you feel you are missing important information, or meet with the instructor to ask further questions.

Tape-recording lectures is another method of ensuring that you are not missing critical points (Meltzer and Palau, 1997). First, however, ask your instructor for permission, as some colleges and/or individual faculty have policies forbidding this practice. Other advantages to taping class lectures include the opportunity to review the lecture repeatedly and the ability to fill in gaps in your notes. If you have a long commute to school, listening to taped lectures is a productive use of this time.

Finally, set aside time each day on your calendar to review lecture material, whether you are preparing for a test, writing a paper, or doing assigned readings for the next class. If you wait several days after a class session before looking back over class notes, you will begin to forget new material. Review class notes periodically, rather than waiting until you begin to study for an exam.

If you feel that despite preparing thoroughly for class, you are not performing as well as you would like, consider studying with a group or seeking help from a tutor. You are *not* in a nursing program all on your own. You have classmates who are experiencing the same concerns and having the same troubles. Sometimes, just getting together with two or three other students for a snack and going over class notes is beneficial. As you increase your knowledge, you also help someone else learn (Nugent and Vitale, 1997).

Most colleges have tutors available for various subjects, and your course instructor can usually direct you to the appropriate resources. Occasionally, an upper class nursing student or faculty member is willing to mentor and/or tutor students who are having difficulty. Do not be shy or too embarrassed to ask for help.

Test-Taking

The best way to alleviate test anxiety is to be thoroughly prepared before going into the test (Meltzer and Palau, 1997). About a week before the exam, begin gathering together any class notes and other materials related to the material to be tested. Set aside time each day to review these materials, comparing the points covered with the same items in the textbook. Make notes on any remaining questions you may have, and allow time to talk with the instructor or classmates for clarification before the day of the exam.

Practice test questions related to the material to be tested. Most textbooks have review questions at the end of each chapter, and many come with computer disks that contain questions. Supplemental questions and activities are also available in student workbooks that accompany the textbook.

Practicing test questions is beneficial for the following reasons: (1) The student develops a sense of comfort in taking exam questions, (2) proficiency in choosing the correct answer improves, and (3) review of right and wrong rationale serves as an effective study technique (Nugent and Vitale, 1997).

The evening before the exam should not be spent cramming. If you have spread your study time out over several days, you should have a fairly good grasp of the content. Eat a balanced meal for dinner, review the material one more time, and get at least seven to eight hours of sleep. If you feel you need to look at your notes once more before the exam, eat a light but nourishing breakfast and allow about an hour for a final review before going to class.

Keep in mind the following suggestions for exams:

1. Lay out all the necessary supplies for the exam—pencils, paper, and a calculator—the night before. You do not need the added stress of attempting to gather these things at the last minute.
2. Make sure you have all the pages to the exam. Count the questions and estimate how much time it will take to answer each one.
3. Read all directions carefully before beginning to answer questions. Make sure your name and/or identifying number is on your answer sheet.
4. Do not panic if you feel that you do not know the answer to the first several questions. This is a common occurrence, as your stress level is high as you begin the exam. Try skipping the first ten questions and going back to them later. This is a technique that is sometimes helpful. Close your eyes, take a few deep breaths, then proceed.
5. Read each question carefully, including the stem and all choices. Avoid the impulse to choose the answer that looks best until you have carefully considered all choices, using the following guidelines:
   a. Cover the answers while reading each question; underline key words and ask yourself what the question is really asking—think about the right answer before reading the choices, then check to see if your answer is present.
   b. Eliminate wrong answers by marking through them—look for obviously incorrect choices first, then try to find the one closest to your answer.
   c. Consider priority answers first—for example, if asked what to do first in a client care situation, consider using the ABCs of CPR or Maslow's hierarchy of basic needs (chapter 4) to prioritize care.
   d. Try to avoid choosing answers containing words such as "always," "never," "all," or "none"—they are often used to distract from the correct answer.
   e. When a selection is made, reread the question to see if the choice fits with it grammatically.
   f. Ask yourself if your choice makes sense—for example, if the question asks for a nursing intervention, be sure you choose an intervention.
6. Choose your answer based on what you have read in the textbook and discussed in class. If you have had previous nursing experience, you'll have a tendency to base your answer on what you would do as an LPN, which may not be correct in this instance.
7. Mark your answer carefully on the answer sheet, making sure it corresponds with the correct number on the exam. Be sure to write neatly and legibly. Answer all short answer and essay questions as completely as possible (more is usually better than not enough).

8. Do not go back and change answers unless you are ABSOLUTELY sure of yourself. Frequently, students who change answers were correct the first time, and suffer as a result of second-guessing themselves.
9. Do not read too much into the questions. Do not assume the instructor is attempting to trick you. Take each question at face value and answer to the best of your ability.
10. After completing the exam, erase stray marks on the answer sheet and make sure you have answered each question.

Once the exam is over, you'll want to know how well you've done. If the instructor goes over the questions, make sure you take advantage of that time to learn anything you have missed. Tests are not intended to penalize students or weed them out. Try to think of an exam as an opportunity—it lets you evaluate what you have learned and identify areas of weakness. Make an appointment to discuss your exam results with the instructor if you haven't done well, or if you have further questions. Approach the instructor in a mature manner, rather than one that is aggressive and attacking. If you disagree about test answers, come prepared to defend your position with books, notes, and other needed materials. Try to make an exam a true learning experience rather than a major stressor.

Academic concerns, time management, and finances are but a few of the day-to-day worries of the returning adult student. Unfortunately, students frequently overlook available resources for help and neglect self-care strategies. You have invested a great deal of time and money in furthering your education. Take care of that investment by following some of the simple strategies mentioned here in order to improve your chances for success.

CRITICAL THINKING EXERCISES

1. Review the background material on Maria, Kevin, and Suzanna in chapter 1 (Box 1–1). Which ones are nontraditional learners? Why? Is any one of the three a traditional student? Why? How could study sessions be organized to meet the needs of each?

_____

_____

_____

_____

_____

_____

_____

2. Using the time management grid below, fill in your activities for one week. Be sure to include time for recreation and rest. Bring the results to class to share with classmates and faculty. How much time are you devoting to studying? Is it enough? Is there wasted time that could be spent more productively?

Time Management Grid

	Sun.	Mon.	Tues.	Wed.	Thurs.	Fri.	Sat.
7AM							
8AM							
9AM							
10AM							
11AM							
12 Noon							
1PM							
2PM							
3PM							
4PM							
5PM							
6PM							
7PM							
8PM							
9PM							
10PM							

*Use the following key to fill in the grid:

Z= Sleep   S= Study
W= Work   R= Recreation
C= Class/Clinical H= Household duties

3. Discuss various strategies that could be used to reduce stress in the LPN/
    LVN who is attending college for the first time.

    _____

    _____

    _____

    _____

    _____

    _____

4. Analyze your personal study habits. Discuss four strategies that could im-
    prove your chances for academic success.

    _____

    _____

    _____

    _____

    _____

    _____

REFERENCES

Bradshaw, M., and K. Nugent (1997). Clinical learning experiences of nontraditional age nursing students. *Nurse Educator* 22(6):40, 47.

Copp, L. (1995). Respecting the nontraditional student. *Journal of Professional Nursing* 11(2):65–66.

deWit, S. (1999). *Saunders student nurse planner: A guide to success in nursing school* (Version 2). Philadelphia: W.B. Saunders.

Hinds, C., B. Malenfant, and A. Home (1995). Balancing family, work and school. *Canadian Nurse* 9:53, 55.

Meltzer, M., and S. Palau (1997). *Learning strategies in nursing: Reading, studying and test-taking* (2nd ed.). Philadelphia: W.B. Saunders.

Nugent, P., and B. Vitale (1997). *Test success: Test-taking techniques for beginning nursing students* (2nd ed.). Philadelphia: F.A. Davis.

Selye, H. (1978). On the real benefits of eustress (interview by Laurence Cherry). *Psychology Today* 11(10):60–70.

Snyder, B. (1992). Adult students: Who are we and what do we need? *Liberal Education* 78(4):46–48.

Warner, C., and N. Dishner (1997). Creating a learning community for adult undergraduate students. *Journal of College Student Development* 38(5):542-543.

Zerwekh, J., and J. Claborn (1999). *Nursing today: Transitions and trends* (3rd ed.). Philadelphia: W.B. Saunders.

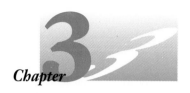

Chapter

Nursing: Past and Present Influences

LEARNING OBJECTIVES

After completing this chapter, you will be able to:

1. Discuss the importance of Florence Nightingale's contributions to modern nursing.
2. Compare and contrast differences in the educational preparation of graduates from associate degree, diploma, and baccalaureate degree nursing programs.
3. Discuss the relevance of the development of professional nursing organizations to the continued growth of the nursing profession.
4. Explain the importance of self-regulation and licensure to the nursing profession.
5. Describe the impact made upon the nursing profession by managed care and merging health care services.
6. Discuss the role of nursing in quality improvement of client care.
7. Describe at least three ways in which future trends in health care will affect nursing practice.

KEY TERMS

Advanced Practice Nurses

Alexian Brothers

American Association of Colleges of Nursing

American Nurses' Association

Clara Barton

Mary Breckenridge

Brown Report

Continuous Quality Improvement

Dorothea Dix

Hotel Dieu

Lavinia Dock

Knights Hospitalers of St. John of Jerusalem

Knights of Saint Lazarus

Managed Care

Mildred Montag

National Council of State Boards of Nursing

National League for Nursing

National Student Nurses' Association

NCLEX-PN

NCLEX-RN

Florence Nightingale

Mary Adelaide Nutting

Linda Richards

Isabel Hampton Robb

Lillian Wald

 Maria, Kevin, and Suzanna are meeting at a local coffee shop to study for an upcoming exam.

Suzanna: I'm so glad we decided to use personal planners to help organize our study time. It really helps me to be able to see where I need to be each day and what I need to be studying to keep up in class.

Maria: Yes, the planner does help. My only problem is, I don't have enough time to complete my schoolwork each day and still be a wife and mother. Last night I tried to read the material for our class on how nursing has evolved, but my husband wanted to discuss our household budget. It's so frustrating sometimes when I can't put in my allotted study time!

Kevin: How about if we finish looking over this microbiology material about fifteen minutes earlier than we planned? Then we can review the information Maria didn't get to last night. It'll help us all to be prepared for class today. I've got to admit, there's a lot to learn about how nursing has changed over time.

F rom the time of the ancient folk healers to that of the present-day nurse practitioner, nursing's history is rich with change (Figure 3–1). The earliest documented nursing organization was formed in 1099 during the First Crusade (1095–1099). Known as the Knights Hospitalers of St. John of Jerusalem, this organization's members provided hospitality and care to thousands of pilgrims and crusaders in the Holy Land (Kalisch and Kalisch, 1995).

1800–1900
Theodor Fliedner organized Deaconess school in Kaiserwerth

Florence Nightingale developed a nursing curriculum based on nursing arts, a combination of nursing theory and practice

Crimean, Civil War & Spanish American War created a need for educated nurses

500–1000
Nursing assigned to women in household and religious orders

1100–1300
Protestant reformation caused nursing care to decline along with the reduction in Catholic religious orders

Three schools of nursing are founded: Bellview, Connecticut, Boston

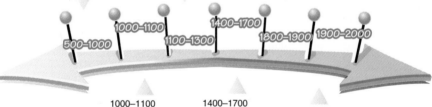

1000–1100
Military influence with the Knights Hospitalers of St. John

1400–1700
Medical advances of vaccinations and pasteurizations

1900–2000
Licensure laws for nursing

WWI and WWII had nurse corps

Clara Barton established the Red Cross

Isabell Hampton Robb founded nursing program at John Hopkins

Yale founds the first university setting for nursing education

Lavinia Dock founded NLN

Lillian Wald founder of first public health nursing service in US

Nursing organizations flourished

Advanced nursing degrees are recognized

Figure 3–1
The evolution of nursing.

During the Middle Ages, the majority of nursing care was performed by religious orders. Later, nursing care became more secular and more structured. Formal training programs were begun, such as that at the Deaconess Institute at Kaiserwerth, Germany, established in 1836.

Influenced by social and political forces and driven by inadequate health care for the hospitalized, Florence Nightingale, a graduate of the Kaiserwerth program, revolutionized the manner in which nurses cared for clients. She instituted changes that affected client survival rates, made nursing more appealing as a profession to young women, and profoundly affected modern-day nursing.

During the early 1980s, the nature of health care began changing dramatically as cost reduction and quality improvement issues surfaced. Shorter hospital stays have forced clients back to the community for completion of care, and nurses have refocused nursing care planning on meeting client-expected outcomes as quickly as possible. Managed care has become a reality, and has affected the way in which clients can access the health care system.

As you obtain registered nurse licensure and take on greater responsibilities, you will be facing increasingly difficult challenges. Now, in the twenty-first century, we are again beginning to experience a nursing shortage. Fewer young people are seeking careers in nursing, largely because of increasingly attractive jobs in high-tech areas, which promise better benefits and less stress.

As a new graduate entering the workforce, you need to be aware of past influences that have shaped nursing, as well as the nature of the present health care environment. This chapter takes you through a brief history of nursing, emphasizing religious, social, and political aspects of nursing's development as a profession. Factors affecting nursing practice in today's world will be explored, as will the development of professional nursing organizations and regulation of practice and licensure.

HISTORICAL FOUNDATIONS

The history of nursing can be traced to the modern day by examining societal influences that shaped the development of the profession. Religious, social, and political factors have all contributed to nursing's history.

Religious

In the West, the establishment of Christianity coincided with the development of groups organized to help care for the sick, orphans, widows, the elderly, and the poor in the name of charity (Kalisch and Kalisch, 1995). Throughout history, nursing has been considered a calling by many—a special vocation in which an individual gives selflessly to others. Hard work, dedication to duty, and benevolence are basic religious values that many denominations honor, and these are the principles upon which nursing began.

Despite the fact that nursing has been a predominantly female profession, males in religious orders took an active part in early care of the sick. The **Knights of Saint Lazarus** (established about 1200) dedicated themselves to caring for people with leprosy, syphilis, and other socially unacceptable diseases (Donahue, 1996). The Knights of Saint John of Jerusalem were members of a male organization who provided care to travelers pursuing spiritual goals. During the bubonic plague epidemic of 1348, another male nursing group, the **Alexian Brothers**, was founded and continues to exist today in dual spiritual/nursing roles.

Benedictine monasteries organized medical schools, some of which afforded female deaconesses the opportunity to pursue a program of study in caring for the sick. In this way, women were able to satisfy intellectual and spiritual aspirations while contributing to the needs of others (Nutting and Dock, 1935). By joining a religious order, unmarried women were given the freedom to provide a service to others outside their own families.

Apart from formal religious orders, some groups of women joined together to care for the sick outside the bounds of the cloister or convent. One such group was the Beguines of Flanders, Belgium. This group was a religious association established in the twelfth century, but its members took no monastic vows. Members, or "sisters", received their preparation to care for others as apprentices under the guidance of more experienced Beguines. They devoted themselves to the needs of widows and orphans of the Crusaders. One of the most famous Beguine hospitals is the **Hotel Dieu** in Paris. Besides working in the hospital, the Beguine sisters also cared for people in their homes (Dolan, Fitzpatrick, and Herrmann, 1983).

The Renaissance, which began in the fourteenth and fifteenth centuries and peaked in the sixteenth and seventeenth centuries, saw a decline in the influence of religious orders, helped along by the emergence of the Protestant Reformation in Europe and England. With these transformations, nursing care, too, saw significant secularizing changes. It has continued to move more fully into the general population, and is no longer primarily the province of religious orders. In our own era, however, we have seen a renewed interest in returning nursing care to the church. During the past several years, parish nursing has achieved a certain popularity. Many churches have instituted parish nursing as a service for their parishioners. The duties of the parish nurse vary with each church organization, but may include visiting the ill, health teaching, and wellness screening for members. Parish nurses provide holistic health care to a faith community (Bergquist and King, 1994).

Social

Perhaps the major social factor affecting the development of nursing is society's attitude toward the role of women. Traditionally, women have been expected to assume the role of wife and mother, tending primarily to their immediate families' needs. Following the Reformation, hospital nursing was often carried out by the "undesirables" of society, such as criminals and prostitutes (Donahue, 1996). They were poorly educated and were described as being drunken and abusive to clients.

With the establishment of the first real school of nursing at Kaiserswerth, Germany, many young women were better educated and more fully prepared to improve nursing care. Perhaps the most famous graduate of this school was **Florence Nightingale** (Figure 3–2).

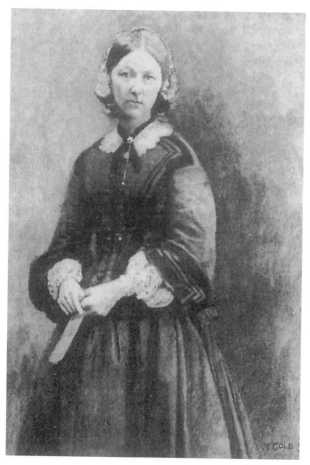

Figure 3-2
Florence Nightingale.

Born into a wealthy family, Florence Nightingale (1820–1910) was highly educated and had social standing in England. Victorian English attitudes of the time supported the belief that gentlewomen should not work outside the home. But, rebelling against her parents' wishes, she received training to become a nurse.

When she learned of the lack of medical and nursing care for British troops during the Crimean War (1853–1856), Nightingale organized a group of 38 nurses to travel to the Crimea in southern Russia. Despite societal opposition, she and her team reached the Crimean battlefields in 1854. They found over-crowding in the hospitals, no medical supplies, and limited space for the sick and injured. Using her own funds, Nightingale obtained supplies, cleaned up the unsanitary conditions, and established laundries to wash linens.

At the end of six months, Nightingale and her nurses had decreased the death rate from 42% to 2% (Dolan et al., 1983). Working long hours to care for casualties of the war, Florence Nightingale was observed many nights making rounds through the battlefields with a lighted lantern, earning her the nickname "the Lady with the Lamp". For her tireless efforts, she was recognized and praised by her countrymen both in the Crimea and in England.

Upon her return home, Florence Nightingale was given a monetary award by the British people. With this money, she established a school of nursing at London's St. Thomas's Hospital in 1860. Again, she was met with opposition from members of society who believed women should remain in the home to care for their own family members (Kalisch and Kalisch, 1995). Nevertheless, the school prospered, largely because of Nightingale's reputation. She was the first woman to be awarded the British Order of Merit, which she received in 1907.

Florence Nightingale's school of nursing emphasized health of the body and soul (Dolan et al., 1983). Nightingale believed that nursing was an art—an art that required organized, practical, and scientific training. She resisted the idea that nurses were to be servants of physicians or any other health care profession-als. Florence Nightingale supported the idea that nurses should be educated to possess a unique body of knowledge that is nursing.

In her book, *Notes on Nursing*, published in 1860, Nightingale defined nursing as "that care which puts a person in the best possible condition for nature to restore or to preserve health, and to prevent or to cure disease or injury". Upon her death, she left contributions in the areas of nursing process, education, theory, and research. Through Nightingale's efforts, nursing gradually came to be viewed as a profession for women of all social levels.

Nineteenth-century attitudes toward women in America were similar to those in England and Europe. But throughout that century, characterized by the Industrial Revolution, women continued to push past societal boundaries to improve nursing education and client care. In 1900, Clara Barton (1821–1912)—the "Angel of the Battlefield" during the American Civil War (1861–

1865)—organized the American Red Cross, which she headed until 1904. In the early twentieth century two other women were of particular importance: **Lillian Wald** (1867–1940), who established a visiting nursing service for poor tenement families in New York City, and **Mary Breckenridge** (1881–1965), who organized a frontier nurses organization in rural Kentucky, which is still in operation today.

As the public began to recognize the benefits of better trained nurses, courtesy of Florence Nightingale's efforts in England, nursing schools began to spring up in the United States. Nursing was becoming more attractive as a vocation for young women. **Linda Richards** (1841–1930), known as America's first trained nurse, worked many years to help improve nursing education. Other contributors to nursing education in America were **Isabel Hampton Robb** (1860–1910), who reduced working hours of students and promoted licensure exams, and **Mary Adelaide Nutting** (1858–1948), who wrote a book on the history of nursing.

The transition to the twentieth century in the United States brought new rights and freedoms for women, together with more recognition of their place in the working world. **Lavinia Dock** (1858–1956) was a well-known nurse who fought for women's rights issues and for the right to vote. Education for nurses became established at universities, and **Mildred Montag** promoted creation of the associate degree as a shorter route into nursing. Medical advances created new ethical concerns and nurses developed professional organizations.

Political

Religious orders, lay people, and soldiers, all have been called upon to provide assistance during times of political conflict throughout history. Whatever the reason, from territorial advancement to the preservation of personal freedoms, societies have waged wars in which nurses have been needed to care for the injured and their families. In fact, many important contributions to the development of professional nursing have been made during times of conflict.

While Florence Nightingale struggled to improve health care in England, Americans, North and South, were fighting the Civil War. Care of the injured was just as disorganized and unsanitary on Union and Confederate battlefields as it was in Europe. Several religious orders responded to the call for efficient, effective nursing care, yet more nurses were needed. Many women who had no formal nursing education volunteered to help.

One such woman was **Dorothea Dix** (1802–1887), a Boston schoolteacher who had been crusading to improve care of the mentally ill in institutions. Appointed superintendent of the Female Nurses of the [Union] Army, Dix organized a training program for women volunteers who met strict criteria, both in moral character and looks (Dix insisted that nurses should be "plain", i.e., unattractive). At the end of a month-long training program, the women qualified to supervise care of the wounded during the Civil War. In the South, however, society continued to frown on women who worked outside the home. Therefore, the wounded were cared for by women in their own homes or by volunteers in hospitals.

The Spanish-American War of 1898 marked the first time trained nurses were accepted in military hospitals. By the outbreak of World War I (1913–1918), both the Army and the Navy had implemented a nurse corps. The Army School of Nursing was formed in 1918 to meet the rising need for nurses to care for battle casualties (Dolan et al., 1983).

During World War II (1939–1945), significant treatment advances helped bring about a higher level of client care. Antibiotics, blood transfusions, and immunizations improved survival rates. Trauma care and rehabilitation became a means of saving and restoring lives. Nurses were involved in all aspects of care, whether in military hospitals, on battleships, or flying on medical evacuation planes.

In the last half of the twentieth century, nurses continued to assist the sick and wounded during the Korean conflict, the Vietnam War, and Operation Desert Storm. Today, nurses serve in various branches of the military as staff nurses, educators, and administrators.

THE EVOLUTION OF NURSING EDUCATION

As we have learned, nursing education has changed from folk medicine, which was passed down through the generations, to formal training programs in hospitals, community colleges, and universities. Today, we see many levels of nursing education: practical (vocational in some states), diploma, associate degree, baccalaureate degree, masters degree, and doctoral degree (Figure 3–3).

Practical/Vocational Nursing

In the early 1900s, the first class for formal training of nurses who would provide "practical" nursing was offered at the YWCA in Brooklyn, New York (Hill and Howlett, 2001). The focus of practical/vocational nursing education was to prepare nurses to care for the elderly, the chronically ill, and sick children in the home. Early training programs were three months long, and included "cooking, care of the house, dietetics, simple science, and simple nursing procedures" (Hill and Howlett, 2001, p.11). During both World Wars, practical/vocational nurses worked in clinics, health departments, industries, and hospitals. By 1962, approximately 60% of working nurses were practical/vocational nurses.

Today, length of education and scope of practice distinguish practical/vocational nurses from registered nurses. Generally, practical/vocational nursing

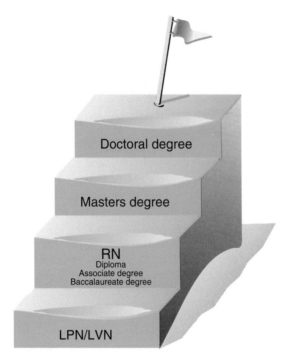

Figure 3–3
Levels of nursing education.

programs are about one year in duration, with classes taking place in vocational/ technical schools, community colleges, and high schools. Graduates must pass the **NCLEX-PN** exam for licensure. The scope of practical/vocational nursing includes meeting basic client needs in hospitals, long-term care facilities, and in the community. Licensed practical/vocational nurses practice under the supervision of a registered nurse or physician.

Career mobility for the practical/vocational nurse is available by "bridging" to the RN level through an LPN/LVN to RN nursing program. The majority of such programs offer an associate degree in nursing to the LPN/LVN after about one year of studies; however, a number of bridge programs for LPN/ LVNs offer a baccalaureate degree (Redmond, 1997). Both types of bridge programs accept coursework from the practical/vocational nursing program, so subject matter is not repeated. With a large number of LPN/LVNs in the nursing workforce and the need for nurses who can care for more complex clients, many practical/vocational nurses are choosing to enter bridge programs to become RNs.

Diploma Nursing

The first type of nursing education program for registered nurses in the United States was the hospital-based diploma school. Students frequently lived in quarters adjacent to the hospital, and were scheduled to work long hours on the client units before or after classroom lectures. Physicians gave many of the lectures, and clinical training was supervised by head nurses. Most programs were two to three years in duration, with students receiving a diploma in nursing upon graduation and being eligible to take the licensure exam for RNs.

Currently, the number of diploma schools has dramatically declined, as education for nurses has moved into a collegiate setting. From 1970 to 1996, the number of new graduates from diploma programs declined from 22,554 to 7049 (McBride, 1999). Diploma schools still exist in some states, however, and continue with a strong emphasis on bedside nursing and clinical skills.

RN to BSN articulation programs are available at many universities, offering diploma and associate degree graduates a means to obtain a baccalaureate degree without repeating basic nursing coursework. Many diploma graduates have discovered the need to obtain a baccalaureate degree in nursing in order to advance in their profession.

Associate Degree Nursing

The associate degree in nursing is the newest form of basic entry into practice as an RN. Based on the research of Dr. Mildred Montag (1951), who was looking for a way to remedy a post–World War II nursing shortage, this type of nursing preparation is about two years in duration and is usually offered at community colleges. Some universities offer "two-plus-two" programs, in which students complete two years toward an associate degree, then return for two more years to receive a baccalaureate degree in nursing.

In 1995, the majority of all basic nursing programs were associate degree in nature (National League for Nursing, 1995). The number of graduates from associate degree in nursing programs in 1996 was almost double that of graduates from diploma and baccalaureate programs (McBride, 1999).

The popularity of the two-year associate degree in nursing stems primarily from its short duration, the part-time and evening study options available at many colleges, and low tuition costs. This type of degree is especially attractive to the nontraditional student or the student with a previous degree, for they can be working as an RN in a shorter period of time than if attending a baccalaureate degree program. Graduates take the same **NCLEX-RN** exam for licensure as diploma and baccalaureate graduates.

Baccalaureate Degree Nursing

In 1948, a report written by Esther Lucille Brown, later called the **Brown Report**, recommended that basic schools of nursing be placed in universities and colleges, and that minorities and men be recruited into nursing. As this idea took hold, the American Nurses' Association (ANA) published a position paper entitled *Educational Preparation for Nurse Practitioners and Assistants to Nurses* (1965).

While preparing this report, the ANA studied nursing care and education, and concluded that the baccalaureate degree in nursing should be the entry point into professional practice. The associate degree level of nursing, according to the paper, is a technical level of practice. The ANA further recommended separate licensure for professional (baccalaureate) and technical (diploma and associate degree) levels of nursing.

This position paper sparked considerable controversy, as the majority of nursing programs of the time were diploma and associate degree in nature. The debate continues to rage over the issue of two levels of nursing practice, since political maneuvering has prevented a resolution. At this time, we continue to have one licensure exam for registered nurses, and one level of licensure, regardless of basic preparation toward registered nursing.

Baccalaureate nursing programs are usually four years long, and consist of general studies courses with a focus in nursing. Students enrolled in a baccalaureate program find a stronger emphasis on leadership, research, and community nursing than those in other nursing programs. Baccalaureate graduates are prepared to practice in a variety of settings, and take the same NCLEX-RN exam as graduates from other programs.

Masters Degree Nursing

Ongoing changes in health care are requiring nurses to be better educated in order to manage the complexities of client care. As care moves to the community, nurses need better critical thinking skills, more sophisticated clinical judgment, advanced assessment skills, and the ability to function independently (Nichols, 1997). Nurses with advanced degrees, or **advanced practice nurses,** will be needed in increasing numbers in the twenty-first century to conduct research into cost containment interventions, serve as consultants, educate future nurses, and direct client care at health care agencies.

The masters degree in nursing is the first level of graduate education for nurses. To obtain a masters in nursing, baccalaureate graduates complete a program of study that varies from two to five years, depending on the amount of coursework taken each semester or quarter. The majority of masters students choose part-time study in order to continue working in current nursing positions. Many universities offer an RN to MSN option, wherein baccalaureate nursing students may complete coursework toward a masters during the course of their basic program.

Students choose a particular area of interest, such as nurse practitioner, nurse educator, clinical specialist, nurse administrator, nurse midwife, or nurse anesthetist. Further specialization is also possible within each of these roles. For example, students may specialize in such areas as family health, adult health, women's health, pediatrics, geriatrics, community health, or mental health.

Masters-prepared nurses are found working in hospitals as nurse administrators and managers, as clinical specialists for a particular population of clients, and as case managers of care. In the community, these advanced practice nurses function as nurse practitioners, coordinate client care in home health agencies, and supervise care in public health clinics. Other masters-level nurses teach nursing students in community college and university settings.

Doctoral Degree Nursing

The doctoral degree is the terminal degree in nursing; it prepares nurses to become faculty members in universities, deans of schools of nursing, vice presidents of hospitals, researchers, and nursing theorists (Nichols, 1997). With an emphasis on nursing theory development and research, the doctorate in nursing is becoming more available to nurses as new programs open across the country.

In 1932, the first student at Columbia University's Teachers College completed her doctoral degree in education with a major in nursing education. Since that time, increasing numbers of nurses have received doctorates in nursing and related fields, such as education, anthropology, sociology, psychology, and biology. The majority of doctoral students are nursing faculty from colleges and universities, who require the degree for promotion and tenure; however, many are administrators of health care agencies and nurse researchers.

The Future of Nursing Education

As nursing moves into the twenty-first century, it is important to understand several changes that will affect the way nurses need to be educated. First, nursing care will be provided at the client's side, wherever that might be. The days of clients' checking into the hospital for two weeks until their symptoms have subsided are long gone. Cost containment and quality care issues will force nurses to take client care to clinics, homes, schools, and churches. Nursing education will shift from agency-based care to client-centered care.

Nursing care will focus on expected client outcomes, rather than nursing interventions. The nursing process (chapter 7) has been the frame upon which client care is based, and will continue to serve this purpose. However, there will be a greater emphasis on planning achievable outcomes, implementing cost-effective measures to meet those outcomes within a given timeframe, and evaluating the effectiveness of care.

Nurses will become more involved in teaching clients about health promotion, instructing in self-care strategies, and in designing population-based health programs (McBride, 1999). Post-baccalaureate nursing education will be more available in order for nurses to learn the necessary skills for these tasks. Nurses will be needed at all levels of client care—health prevention and promotion, health restoration, and rehabilitation.

Finally, nurses must be more prepared to individualize care to the particular population or culture they serve. Nursing students have become more diverse in terms of age, race, gender, and culture. This diversity is bringing a wider segment of the population into nursing and will, we hope, provide clients with more nurses who are sensitive to individual differences and health care needs.

THE DEVELOPMENT OF PROFESSIONAL NURSING ORGANIZATIONS

At the end of the nineteenth century, the education of nurses was as varied as the many settings in which it took place. Although nurses were beginning to be recognized as trained members of the health care team, they had not yet united to share knowledge and define a common purpose. Nursing leaders, such as Isabel Hampton Robb, understood that nurses could accomplish more as a group than as individuals. The founders of present-day nursing organizations shared common concerns regarding standardization of nursing education and the protection of the public from inadequate nurses (Piemonte and Redman, 1997).

In 1893, Robb helped establish the American Society of Superintendents of Training Schools for Nurses of the United States and Canada, the first nursing organization in the United States (Ellis and Hartley, 1995). This organization, known today as the **National League for Nursing** (NLN), was originally formed to provide standards of education upon which nursing programs should be based, and has retained this purpose into the twenty-first century.

The primary function of the National League for Nursing has been accreditation of all types of schools of nursing. However, the organization also presents workshops and seminars, offers consultation to schools seeking to improve their curricula, and provides evaluation and testing services. In 1995, the NLN announced a strategic plan to focus on community-based health care education and health care delivery. Accreditation is also possible for baccalaureate nursing programs through the **American Association of Colleges of Nursing** (AACN).

A second nursing organization, the **American Nurses' Association** (ANA), was also formed because of the efforts of Isabel Hampton Robb. The ANA is currently recognized as the professional organization for American registered nurses. Established in 1896, the ANA originally contained members from the United States and Canada; however, Canadian members later formed a separate organization. Registered nurses become members of the ANA by joining State Nurse Associations (SNAs).

As its primary purposes, the ANA seeks to "foster high standards of nursing practice, to promote the welfare of nurses, and to improve the general working conditions of nurses" (Donahue, 1996, p. 325). Activities of the ANA include policy-making, specialty area certification for members, and representation of nurses in legislative and collective bargaining matters. The ANA also produces a large variety of educational materials for nurses.

The **National Student Nurses' Association** (NSNA), formed in 1952, is the professional organization for nursing students. This organization has close ties to the ANA; however, the NSNA is a separate association that is run totally

BOX 3-1 *A Sample Listing of Nursing Organizations in the United States*

American Nurses' Association
American Academy of Nurse Practitioners
American Assembly for Men in Nursing
American Association for the History of Nursing
American Association of Colleges of Nursing
American Association of Critical Care Nurses
American Association of Neuroscience Nurses
American Association of Nurse Anesthetists
American College of Nurse Midwives
American Nephrology Nurses' Association
American Organization of Nurse Executives
American Psychiatric Nurses' Association
American Society of Post Anesthesia Nurses
Association of Nurses in AIDS Care
Association of Operating Room Nurses
Association of Rehabilitation Nurses
Association of Women's Health, Obstetric and Neonatal Nurses
Emergency Nurses Association
Hospice Nurses Association
Intravenous Nurses Society
National Association of Orthopedic Nurses
National Association of School Nurses
National Black Nurses Association
National Flight Nurses Association
National Gerontological Nurses Association
National League for Nursing
National Organization for the Advancement of Associate Degree Nursing
National Student Nurses' Association
Sigma Theta Tau

by student nurses. Individual nursing programs send delegates to the NSNA. Representatives of the NSNA may serve on selected committees of the ANA, and give input regarding nursing student issues. Participation in NSNA gives students an opportunity to begin the professional socialization process.

Nursing organizations are formed for many reasons; however, the advancement of nursing and the promotion of quality nursing care form common threads among them. The National League for Nursing and American Nurses' Association have significantly empowered nurses in their profession. Unfortunately, many practicing nurses do not participate in nursing organizations because of busy schedules, the relatively high membership dues, and a concern that nurses' daily problems are not addressed (Nelson, 1997). More often, nurses are choosing to join specialty organizations with which they can more readily identify, such as the National Organization for the Advancement of Associate Degree Nursing (NOAADN), the Emergency Nurses Association, or the Hospice Nurses Association. Box 3–1 contains a partial listing of nursing organizations in the United States. See Appendix B for a more comprehensive list of specialty organizations. The benefits of belonging to professional nursing associations include the development of leadership skills, recognition through certification, legislative lobbying power, access to professional publications, continuing education, and eligibility for insurance (Piemonte and Redman, 1997).

REGULATION OF PRACTICE AND LICENSURE

Despite Florence Nightingale's many contributions to present-day nursing, her vision of how nursing should be did not include registration or licensure. Arguing that nurses should not graduate from a nursing program or receive licensure in their profession, she believed that nurses would then discontinue their educational efforts and stagnate. But her views did not prevail. Today, nursing practice is carefully regulated by each state board of nursing, where the scope of nursing practice and licensure requirements are clearly defined to assure the public of safe practitioners (see chapter 10). Indeed, many states require evidence of continuing education for nurses before approving license renewal.

Since 1944, state boards of nursing have cooperated in the effort to recognize one exam for licensure as a registered nurse. For several years, the ANA had the task of overseeing test question development while the NLN served as the testing service. As of 1978, the **National Council of State Boards of Nursing** (NCSBN) has been responsible for test question development and setting the minimum passing score (Betts, 2001). The exam, once taken by paper and pencil, is now computerized for both RN and LVN/LPN candidates. An emphasis of the computerized adaptive testing (CAT) licensure exam is the measurement of critical thinking and nursing competence.

It is extremely important for nursing to regulate its own licensure and certification, for other professionals do not have the same understanding of the body of knowledge. We must continue to work toward designing exams that will measure nursing knowledge and competence.

When you graduated from your practical/vocational nursing program, you took the NCLEX-PN (National Council Licensure Examination for Practical Nurses). Passing that exam allowed you to apply for licensure in the state where you wanted to work. Graduates from registered nursing programs take the NCLEX-RN; they, too, must make application to the state board of nursing for licensure.

One advantage of a single exam for all licensure candidates is facilitation of licensure by endorsement. This means that a nurse who is practicing in one state may move to another without having to take another licensing exam. By contacting the state board of nursing in the state to which they plan to move, nurses can obtain information as to licensing requirements, which usually include a fee and proof of previous licensure. Each state board of nursing also evaluates potential licensees for infractions against previous licenses before making the decision as to issuance of a license.

Certification of nurses by area of specialty is another function of individual state boards of nursing. This is a credential beyond registered nurse licensure, and includes such groups as Certified Registered Nurse Anesthetists (CRNAs) and Family Nurse Practitioners (FNPs). Certification credentials indicate preparation and expertise beyond a minimum level of nursing education (Nelson, 1997).

As nursing moves into the twenty-first century, you, as a new graduate, will need to be mindful of health care changes that may affect your licensure and practice. The final section of this chapter brings us to where nursing is now, in a climate of economic restrictions and increasing client care complexity.

NURSING TODAY: FACTORS INFLUENCING PRACTICE

The health care system in the United States has undergone many changes since the founding of the initial 13 colonies. Health care has moved from the home to the hospital, and most recently back to the home again. As health education for the public has improved and technology has provided better medications and treatments for most diseases, Americans have enjoyed longer, healthier lives.

Until the early 1980s, most Americans were content to be passive recipients of care in a system that poured millions of dollars into acute care and rehabilitation, with little attention to cost containment and health promotion. As health care costs began to rise to uncontrollable levels, it became apparent that millions of Americans were either uninsured or were rapidly losing the ability to pay for health care (Catalano, 1996).

As you enter the health care environment of today as a registered nurse, you will encounter challenges created by several factors. Client care of the present and future will be affected by the following: (1) an aging population; (2) an emphasis on health maintenance and disease prevention; (3) outcomes-oriented, client-centered care; (4) cost containment; and (5) quality improvement.

It is estimated that by the year 2030, there will be about 65 million older Americans (Campbell, 1997). With this "graying of America" will come an increase in clients with multisystem health care problems and chronic illnesses. The elderly currently utilize more health care dollars per person than do younger members of the American population. They typically have fewer years of schooling, rely heavily on Medicare for financial support, have chronic illnesses, and are widowed. These factors add up to more use of health care resources at a greater cost.

Nurses must respond to a shift in demographics by becoming more knowledgeable in geriatric and home health care (Figure 3–4). More research is needed, for example, in the areas of Alzheimer's disease and other forms of dementia so nurses are better equipped to care for the aged and their families. In the past, the elderly have been placed in nursing homes when they were no longer able to care for themselves. Nursing education programs have emphasized

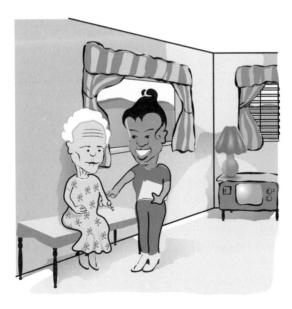

Figure 3–4
Our aging population will demand greater nursing adaptability.

care of hospitalized clients, and have provided most of the clinical experiences for students in such settings rather than in long-term care facilities. As a result, many of today's practicing nurses have not received education specific to geriatric care.

Since hospital stays have been reduced, future nursing education will need to be in settings where the elderly require assistance—the home, neighborhood clinics, churches, and community centers. Psychosocial aspects of aging need to be addressed, as does helping the elderly obtain access to needed resources.

As the general population becomes more involved in maintaining a healthy lifestyle, nurses are taking an active part in client teaching about health promotion and disease prevention. In the past, nurses usually had contact with clients only during an episode of illness or injury. At present, nurses counsel clients about health screening, dietary needs, exercise programs, and treatment regimes for various medical problems. Besides providing care during acute illnesses, nurses are instrumental in teaching clients self-care strategies for discharge home.

With an increased level of knowledge about their own health needs, consumers have become more involved in health care decision making. This has eased the transition into an outcomes-based system of care that is client-centered, since client participation is necessary in order to meet desired goals. As health care costs rise and insurance companies tighten restrictions on services provided, health care professionals are working very closely with clients to set goals that can be achieved as quickly as possible. Through use of the nursing process, nurses help clients develop expected outcomes and plan interventions to achieve the desired results (see chapter 7).

Nurses are working with population groups, as well as individual clients, to develop health-related goals. For example, community health nurses participate in multidisciplinary planning meetings to set outcomes for clients. No matter where the client is within the health care system, nurses are playing an important role in helping achieve positive experiences for clients with minimal complications.

The dominant focus of client care in the current healthcare environment is to contain rising costs. Hospitals, faced with financial difficulties, are merging into large health care systems. **Managed care**, an insurance-based approach to reducing costs, has invaded client care in every setting. Case managers (see chapter 6) coordinate client care activities as the client moves through the health care system.

Terms such as Diagnostic Related Groups (DRGs), Preferred Provider Organizations (PPOs), and Health Maintenance Organizations (HMOs) (Box 3–2) have become commonplace. Consumers, once responsible for paying for their own health care, have become dependent upon third parties in order to be able

Box 3-2 *Health Care Payment Sources*

Medicare—national and state health insurance program for older adults.

Medicaid—federal public assistance program to assist those with financial needs.

Prospective Payment System—limits the amount paid to hospitals that are reimbursed by Medicare; uses Diagnostic Related Groups (DRGs) to establish pretreatment diagnosis billing categories.

Private Insurance—a form of third-party reimbursement. Carried as individual or group coverage through a job; the company pays either a portion or the entire cost.

Health Maintenance Organizations (HMOs)—a group health care agency. A prepaid fee is set without regard to type of treatment. The emphasis is on health maintenance and disease prevention; clients are limited in use of providers and services.

Preferred Provider Organizations (PPOs)—a group of physicians and agencies provides services to employees of a company through an insurance company. In return for using the specified physicians and agencies, clients receive a discounted rate for services.

to afford treatment. Nurses are challenged to deliver quality nursing care in an environment that limits consumers' options. Consider the following questions:

Based on personal experience as a nurse, have you cared for a client for whom you believe the type and amount of provided health care was influenced by his or her ability to pay for services? If so, please describe the circumstances and the outcome for the client:

_____

_____

_____

_____

_____

_____

What, if any, actions were taken by nursing personnel to ensure the best possible care for this client? What do you think could or should have been done differently for this client?

_____

_____

_____

_____

_____

_____

_____

Despite these restrictions, health care systems and clients share a common expectation—quality care. Nurses, who spend more time with clients than other health care professionals, are instrumental in ensuring appropriate, viable care (Malloch and Porter-O'Grady, 1999). What was once called quality assurance in client care is now termed **continuous quality improvement**. This is a process in which the quality of client care is continuously monitored for effectiveness.

The quality of care may be assessed from the time a client enters the health care system until discharge. At each step of the way, all disciplines should be involved in measuring client outcomes against a set of standards that promote excellence. Many organizations utilize clinical care pathways, or care paths as a format for assuring that clients are "on track" to accomplish set goals (see chapter 9). As problems are identified, action should be taken to prevent complications and increased length of stay within the system.

Hospitals and community agencies are employing nurses as outcomes managers, case managers, and quality improvement managers to monitor the quality of client care. By maximizing a client's chances of achieving expected outcomes, costs will be reduced, clients will have fewer complications, and customer satisfaction will be improved.

As we consider nursing in the future, we must be aware of the number of social, economic, and political forces that will influence health care and, ultimately, the type of nursing care needed. The ANA developed a Social Policy Statement (1995) that describes four services expected from nursing:

1. Provision of information and treatment in matters of health and illness.
2. Assistance in resolving problems and managing health-promoting behaviors.

3. Assistance in identifying short- and long-term goals.
4. Acting as an advocate for people dealing with barriers encountered in obtaining health care.

Nurses will be increasingly called upon to assume leadership roles in designing care for vulnerable population groups, in demonstrating quality care, and in cost containment (O'Neil and Coffman, 1998).

We have indeed come a long way from the days of folk healers and untrained volunteers on the battlefield. Nurses have had a colorful, productive history. Let us look eagerly to the future by understanding our past and taking advantage of the opportunities for professional growth that loom on the horizon.

CRITICAL THINKING EXERCISES

1. How have Florence Nightingale's contributions to nursing affected your practice? List three of her beliefs about nursing that you apply to client care.

_____

_____

_____

_____

_____

_____

2. Choose a professional nursing organization to which you would like to belong and describe how you believe membership in the organization would help you grow professionally.

_____

_____

_____

_____

_____

_____

3. Explain the importance of an understanding of present trends in health care to everyday nursing practice.

_____

_____

_____

_____

_____

_____

4. Describe three ways in which an advanced practice nursing degree (masters level or above) would be of benefit in today's changing health care environment.

_____

_____

_____

_____

_____

_____

REFERENCES

American Nurses Association (1965). *Educational preparation for nurse practitioners and assistants to nurses: A position paper* (Publication No. G-83). Kansas City, MO.

Bergquist, S., and J. King (1994). Parish nursing: A conceptual framework. *Journal of Holistic Nursing* 12(2):155–170.

Betts, V. (2001). Legal aspects of nursing. In *Professional nursing: Concepts and challenges* (3rd ed.), K. Chitty, ed. Philadelphia: W.B. Saunders.

Campbell, C. (2001). The social context of nursing. In *Professional nursing: Concepts and challenges* (3rd ed.), K. Chitty, ed. Philadelphia: W.B. Saunders.

Catalano, J. (1996). *Contemporary professional nursing.* Philadelphia: F.A. Davis.

Dolan, J., M. Fitzpatrick, and E. Herrmann (1983). *Nursing in society: A historical perspective* (15th ed.). Philadelphia: W.B. Saunders.

Donahue, M. (1996). *Nursing: The finest art, an illustrated history* (2nd ed.). St. Louis: Mosby-Yearbook.

Ellis, J., and C. Hartley (1995). *Nursing in today's world: Challenges, issues, and trends* (5th ed.). Philadelphia: J.B. Lippincott.

Hill, S., and H. Howlett (2001). *Success in practical nursing: Personal and vocational issues* (4th ed.). Philadelphia: W.B. Saunders.

Kalisch, P., and B. Kalisch (1995). *The advance of American nursing* (3rd ed.). Philadelphia: J.B. Lippincott.

Malloch, K., and T. Porter-O'Grady (1999). Partnership economics: Nursing's challenge in a quantum age. *Nursing Economics* 17(6):299–307.

McBride, A. (1999). Breakthroughs in nursing education: Looking back, looking forward. *Nursing Outlook* 47(3):114–119.

Montag, M. (1951). *The education of nursing technicians.* New York: Putnam.

National League for Nursing (1995). *State approved schools of nursing RN 1995* (Publication No. 19–2689). New York.

Nelson, N. (1997). Image of nursing: Influences of the present. In *Nursing today: Transition and trends* (2nd ed.), J. Zerwekh and J. Claborn, eds. Philadelphia: W.B. Saunders.

Nichols, E. (2001). Educational patterns in nursing. In *Professional nursing: Concepts and challenges* (3rd ed.), K. Chitty, ed. Philadelphia: W.B. Saunders.

Nutting, M., and L. Dock (1935). *A history of nursing.* New York: G.P. Putnam.

O'Neil, E., and J. Coffman (1998). *Strategies for the future of nursing: Changing roles, responsibilities, and employment patterns of registered nurses.* San Francisco: Jossey-Bass.

Piemonte, R., and B. Redman (1997). Professional associations. In *Professional nursing: Concepts and challenges* (2nd ed.), K. Chitty, ed. Philadelphia: W.B. Saunders.

Redmond, G. (1997). LPN-BSN: Education for a reformed health care system. *Journal of Nursing Education* 36(3):121–127.

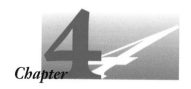

Chapter

Theoretical Foundations of Nursing

LEARNING OBJECTIVES

After completing this chapter, you will be able to:

1. Discuss four concepts basic to most nursing theories.
2. Describe how non-nursing theorists have influenced nursing practice.
3. Explain the importance of theory-guided, research-based nursing practice.
4. Apply selected nursing theories to client care.

Concepts	Health	Philosophies
Conceptual Models	Nursing	Propositions
Environment	Person	Theory

 Maria, Kevin, and Suzanna are walking together to the library where they hope to find material for a written assignment on early nursing leaders.

Kevin: Boy, I never knew so many people influenced nursing. And look at this assignment . . . this list of nursing leaders just seems endless!

Maria: I can see why it's important to understand where we came from . . . it helps us appreciate where we are now as nurses. But why do we have to study about nursing theorists?

Suzanna: I agree, Maria. There's so much to learn about what the signs and symptoms of diseases are and how to interpret client information. Why do we have to learn about what other people think about nursing? Shouldn't nurses with higher degrees concentrate on that? I just want to care for clients right now . . . and to me, that means focusing on the "how to" aspects of nursing.

To be considered a profession, a discipline needs a specialized body of knowledge that sets it apart from other professions (Catalano, 1996). Nursing scholars have directed a great deal of effort toward defining such a body of knowledge—one that will describe what is truly nursing. One such attempt has been in the area of nursing theory development, which began with Florence Nightingale in the nineteenth century and gained momentum in the mid-twentieth century. Today, we have a variety of nursing theories, each offering a slightly different perspective on the nature of nursing.

This chapter presents an introduction to nursing concepts and theories together with their uses in client care, thereby offering you a better understanding of the world of nursing. As a registered nurse, you will be expected to plan holistic nursing care for clients of all ages and cultural backgrounds. Knowledge of the theoretical basis for nursing and the use of non-nursing theories will assist you in analyzing client information from a broader perspective.

WHAT IS NURSING THEORY?

A theory is a general explanation of why something occurs. Theories also attempt to predict, control, and understand phenomena (Massey, 1998). In other words, a theory provides us with a proposed explanation for why certain things happen as they do. For example, Sir Isaac Newton explained the earth's pull on objects in his theory of gravity.

Theories contain concepts, or mental images of data, that are linked by propositions—statements about how two or more concepts are related. For example, *pain* and *anxiety* are concepts that might be found in a nursing theory; and the statement "anxiety has a negative effect on pain" is a proposition linking the concepts of pain and anxiety. Theories are made up of many such propositions (Figure 4–1).

According to Meleis (1997), "Theoretical thinking is essential to all professional undertakings" (p. 8). The complex nature of our present health care system requires nurses to be able to think critically and make decisions that are based on sound scientific principles. Nursing theory is therefore necessary in order for nurses to have a knowledge base upon which to draw for decision making.

Historically, much nursing care has been based on tradition and intuition rather than scientific principles (Upton, 1999). This approach has contributed to a lack of understanding of what nursing really is. In order to set nursing on a firm scientific foundation, research must be conducted to provide a basis for nursing actions.

For many years, nursing research efforts were more often focused on nursing education and administration than on clinical practice. Consequently, a theory–

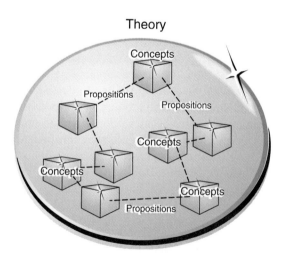

Figure 4–1
The relationship between theory, concepts, and propositions.

practice gap exists, creating confusion over the use of nursing theory in actual practice (Rolfe, 1996). Fortunately, an increase in university-based higher education for nurses has provided more masters and doctorally prepared nurses to lead the effort to conduct client-centered nursing research.

At this time, no one nursing theory has been found to encompass the whole of nursing. Various nursing theorists have suggested explanations as to the relationship between nursing, the client, the environment, and health (four commonly occurring concepts in nursing theories). Portions of these and other theories have been applied to everyday client care.

MAJOR CONCEPTS IN NURSING

Theories attempt to describe concepts of importance to the profession. In nursing, four basic concepts are essential to an understanding of nursing practice:

- Person—the recipient of nursing care; may refer to an individual, family, group, or community; the terms *man*, *patient*, and *client* have also been used.
- Environment—the setting in which nursing care activities take place; also known as the sum of all conditions, influences, and circumstances affecting the person; social, spiritual, and cultural factors are included.
- Health—a dynamic state; may change from day to day; may be viewed as a continuum with high-level wellness at one end and death at the other; the person may move from one point to another as factors affect health.
- Nursing—the diagnosis and treatment of human responses to actual or potential health problems (ANA, 1995); activities and interactions with clients.

A nursing theory, therefore, usually contains most or all of these concepts. Some authors do not include nursing as one of the major concepts. According to Meleis (1997), the inclusion of nursing as a concept would be needless repetition, since the first three help define nursing. However, most nursing theories are analyzed according to their explanations of these four concepts.

SCIENTIFIC THEORIES INFLUENCING NURSING THEORY

As a practical/vocational nursing student, you probably studied several theories of human development, such as Maslow's theory of human motivation and Freud's theory of psychosexual development. In order to understand our discussion of nursing theory, it is important that you be familiar with these and other non-nursing theories that guide us in understanding human behavior. Therefore, a review of selected developmental theories will be included in this discussion, with an emphasis on their application to client care.

Nursing theory development is considered by many to still be in its infancy. In an attempt to develop a common body of nursing knowledge, many nursing theories contain components that have been borrowed from other disciplines. The following are among the most commonly utilized non-nursing theories: systems theory, human needs theory, developmental theory, and stress/adaptation theory.

Leopold von Bertalanffy, a theoretical biologist, first described general systems theory in the late 1930s. He defined a *system* as a set of interrelated components that form a whole. Within a system, each part is essential in making up the whole. The system receives input, produces output, participates in evaluation of success or failure, and supplies feedback to itself. There is a continuous exchange of energy and information between a system and the environment that strives to achieve a balance known as *homeostasis* (von Bertalanffy, 1968).

A human being can easily be compared to the system described in this theory, as can members of a family unit. Systems theory has been used in nursing to describe care given to individuals, families, and communities. Betty Neuman, Sister Callista Roy, and Rosemarie Parse are nursing theorists who have used a systems approach to explain client care.

In 1954, psychologist Abraham Maslow developed a theory of human motivation, which was outlined as a hierarchy of human needs (Figure 4–2). Maslow

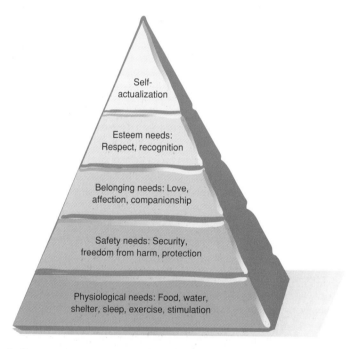

Figure 4–2
Maslow's hierarchy of human needs.

suggests that human behavior is motivated by needs, the most basic being those that must be met to sustain physiological survival—oxygen, food, water, shelter, sleep and rest, and sexual expression. Safety and security needs are on the second level of the hierarchy, and include the need for an environment free from harm. Love and belonging and self-esteem needs are on the next two higher levels, respectively. These involve relational, belonging, and sense-of-self needs. Self-actualization is the highest level, one that Maslow believed few people truly achieve. He maintained that some people have intermittent "peak" experiences at this level during times of great accomplishment; however, continuous attainment of such a level is probably not possible (Maslow, 1954).

The theory suggests that basic needs must be met before higher-level needs become important to the individual. For example, a client in pain would not be motivated to seek new social relationships until the lower level need for comfort is met. Maslow believed that dominant needs that motivate an individual will vary at different points in life (Maslow, 1954). Illness might distract a client from striving toward self-actualization, which requires a person to function at the fullest potential. Human needs theory is used frequently in nursing education to teach students to prioritize client problems.

Several theorists have contributed to the body of knowledge regarding human development. The works of Sigmund Freud and Erik Erikson are two of the most commonly used to describe the behavior of individuals at different stages in life. Both theories suggest that people progress through stages that must be mastered before moving on to the next.

A psychoanalyst, Freud based his theory on the psychosexual development of individuals across the lifespan. He described the mind as consisting of the id, the ego, and the superego. According to Freud, the *id* is concerned mainly with self-gratification without consideration of the consequences. The *ego*, or reality portion of the mind, is the mediator between the id and the *superego*, which is the conscience. Freud's theory consists of psychosexual stages of development in which he categorized people according to age:

Birth to 2 years of age—Oral Stage: Derives pleasure from oral gratification, such as sucking

2 to 4 years of age—Anal Stage: Learns to control excretory functions for gratification

4 to 6 years of age—Phallic Stage: Displays curiosity about genitals; identifies with same-sex parent

6 to 12 years of age—Latency Stage: Focuses on peer relationships; energy directed toward physical and mental growth

12 to 20 years—Genital Stage: Derives pleasure from genital function and heterosexual relationships

This developmental theory has been applied in the nursing care of children and young adults; however, many critics argue that Freud focused excessively on the sexual aspects of development to the exclusion of others (Figure 4–3). Freud described both positive and negative outcomes for each stage. He theorized that all people move through the five stages. As they do so, they experience, confront, and resolve conflicts between the id, ego, and superego along the way. Failure to resolve these conflicts may impede movement through succeeding stages (Craven and Hirnle, 2000). As shown, Freud's stages do not address needs specific to middle-aged and older adults.

Erikson (1950), a developmental psychologist, based his theory of development on Freud's; however, he believed that personality development is also influenced by the social and cultural aspects of society. He explained that development occurs across the lifespan, and that interactions with the environment are instrumental in the formation of a healthy personality. His eight stages of development progress from birth to death, and represent developmental crises that must be mastered before proceeding to the next stage (Table 4–1).

Like Freud, Erikson believed each stage contained positive and negative outcomes. Successful achievement of a positive outcome prepares an individual

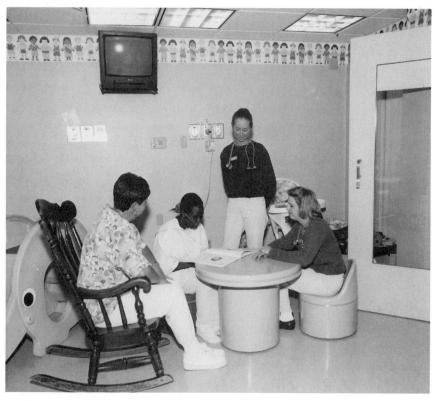

Figure 4–3
Developmental theories help nurses plan care for children.

TABLE 4-1
Erikson's Psychosocial Stages of Development

STAGE	CONFLICT	RESOLUTION
Infant	Trust vs. mistrust	Learns to trust caregivers
Toddler	Autonomy vs. shame and doubt	Gains independence
Preschool	Initiative vs. guilt	Develops self-confidence
School-age	Industry vs. inferiority	Learns to get pleasure from accomplishments
Adolescence	Identity vs. role confusion	Establishment of a sense of identity
Young adult	Intimacy vs. isolation	Develops close personal relationships
Middle adult	Generativity vs. stagnation	Finds satisfying work
Older adult	Ego integrity vs. despair	Finds life to have been fulfilling

for further growth; a negative resolution of a developmental stage interferes
with further development. For example, parents who stifle a three-year-old's
natural tendencies to achieve autonomy may contribute to the child's experiencing feelings of self-doubt as an adult.

This theory is widely used in nursing to assist with planning care appropriate
to the client's developmental level. An understanding of the psychosocial forces
in a client's life helps a nurse to assess for positive or negative resolution of a
particular stage. Consider the following scenario:

> Sarah, a 23-year-old recent college graduate, was diagnosed with leukemia
> and started on chemotherapy four weeks ago. She has severe nausea and
> vomiting, mouth ulcers, and has had a 12-pound weight loss. Sarah is
> scheduled to begin a new teaching job in less than two weeks. Her fiancé
> tells Sarah's nurse that she has become withdrawn and will not talk to him
> when he comes to visit.

Using Maslow's hierarchy of basic human needs, list Sarah's problems in order
of priority:

_____

_____

_____

_____

_____

_____

Within which of Erikson's psychosocial stages of development does Sarah belong? Is she achieving positive or negative resolution of the stage? Why or why not?

_____

_____

_____

_____

_____

_____

Hans Selye's work with human responses to stress has also been used in nursing to explain client behavior. He viewed stress as the body's specific response to any demand made upon it (Selye, 1950). The term *stressor* is used to refer to any nonspecific demand requiring adaptation. Selye theorized that clients experience a *general adaptation syndrome*, which describes a series of phases the body goes through in response to stress (see chapter 8).

According to Selye, the general adaptation syndrome consists of the following stages: (1) the alarm reaction—the body experiences changes to prepare to defend against stressors; (2) the stage of resistance—the body attempts to mobilize resources to cope with stressors; (3) the stage of exhaustion—this occurs if the body is unable to adapt and death ensues. A central theme of Selye's theory is the ability of the person to adapt to stressors, which may be either positive (eustress) or negative (distress).

Stress/adaptation theory may be used in nursing to explain client responses to illness. For example, in the scenario just described, Sarah is experiencing stress related to her illness. The alarm reaction phase for this client occurs early in the illness and consists of both physical and psychological preparation to resist the stressor. During the resistance phase, the client attempts to adapt to the illness. If successful adaptation takes place, the stage of exhaustion will not occur; however, if adaptation energy is exhausted, death is the eventual outcome. In this scenario, Sarah is in the resistance phase, since she is exhibiting symptoms of nausea, vomiting, mouth ulcers, depression, and withdrawal from significant others.

Selye also described specific physiological responses to stress, such as sweating, palpitations, and dilated pupils. In addition to the body's general response to stress, Selye discussed a local response, or local adaptation syndrome, such as that which occurs with local inflammation. He hypothesized that stress plays a role in every disease process, regardless of the cause.

Non-nursing theories from other scientific disciplines provide nurses with predictions as to how humans will behave in particular situations. Since nursing is aimed at holistic client care, it is helpful to use these theories in providing comprehensive client care.

NURSING THEORY AS A BASIS FOR PRACTICE

In the middle of the twentieth century, interest in defining nursing knowledge increased as nurses became aware that theories from other disciplines could not completely describe nursing. As more nurses received graduate-level education, nurse theorists began developing **philosophies** (systems of basic principles) and **conceptual models** (graphic representations of concepts and their relationships) of nursing.

Personal experiences in nursing and education influenced theorists to write about their perceptions of nursing theory (Massey, 1998). With the rise of doctorally prepared nurses, research became the means for gathering data to support theoretical propositions in nursing theories. An increasing number of nursing scholars are working to define nursing's body of knowledge.

Following is a brief discussion of the most commonly recognized nursing theorists and major concepts (italicized) defined in each theory. Table 4–2 provides a listing of selected theorists by theory name and description. A more detailed analysis of each theory may be obtained by further readings from the reference list at the end of the chapter.

Florence Nightingale

Florence Nightingale is considered by many to be the first nursing theorist. She viewed control of the *environment* as extremely important to client care. Nightingale believed that the main purpose of the *nurse* was to provide a service to people and ensure that the *client* (the recipient of care) returned to *health* (a state of well-being) by manipulation of the environment. This was to be accomplished by providing clean air, fresh water, cleanliness, and light (Nightingale, 1860).

Hildegard Peplau

Peplau's theory states that *nursing* is a goal-directed interpersonal process oriented toward assisting clients to meet their needs. The *client* seeks assistance because of perceived needs, and enters into a therapeutic relationship with the nurse. The psychodynamic nature of the relationship is a part of the *environment* in which nursing care is received by the client, as are social and cultural influences (Peplau, 1952). *Health* is viewed as a state in which needs are met and the client experiences personal growth by becoming more creative and productive.

TABLE 4-2
Selected Nursing Theories

THEORIST	THEORY	FOCUS OF THEORY
Nightingale	Environmental	Provide care by manipulating environment to optimize return to health
Peplau	Interpersonal	Interpersonal process between nurse and client assists the client to reduce anxiety and maintain equilibrium
Rogers	Unitary Humanism	Assist client to achieve harmony between energy fields of human and environment
Orem	Self-Care Deficit	Assist to identify and minimize the individual self-care deficit
Roy	Adaptation	Promotion of adaptation and coping to environmental stressors
Neuman	Systems	Assist to identify and minimize the negative effects of the environment to promote equilibrium
Leininger	Culture Care	Assist with health care needs as defined by the client's cultural perception of health
Parse	Humanistic Becoming	Facilitate the changing process of "becoming" as the client includes the health experience as part or the perceived quality of life
Watson	Caring	Health care delivery based on "carative factors" using curative and preventative holistic measures

Martha Rogers

Martha Rogers describes *nursing* as a humanistic science that contains a body of knowledge necessary for practice. The main goal of nursing is the maintenance and return of the client to health. She views *clients* as unitary beings who are irreducible, whole, four-dimensional energy fields. According to Rogers, humans and their *environment* are dynamic, infinite energy fields (Rogers, 1986). *Health and illness* exist on a continuum, and are influenced by harmony or conflict between people and their environment.

Dorothea Orem

Orem's self-care deficit theory focuses on identifying the client's self-care needs and planning nursing interventions to meet those needs. The theory defines the *client* as a biopsychosocial being capable of self-care, but who may have limitations that prevent effective self-care (Orem, 1971). The main goal of *nursing* is to assist with these limitations. The *environment* is made up of internal and external stimuli that affect *health*, which is a state of wholeness or integrity.

Sister Callista Roy

Roy's theory is based on concepts from systems and adaptation theories, wherein the *client* is described as a holistic adaptive system (Roy and Andrews, 1991). Adaptive responses occur in one of four modes: physiological, self-concept, role function, and interdependence. The *environment* encompasses all conditions, circumstances, and influences surrounding and affecting the development of the client. Roy believes *health* is a state and process of being as the person adapts to problems. The main goal of *nursing* is to promote adaptation and coping to environmental stressors.

Betty Neuman

Betty Neuman was also influenced by systems theory, but included components of stress theory in her description of nursing. In her view, *health* exists when all parts of the *person* are in harmony with the *environment*, which consists of internal and external forces surrounding the person at any given time. The client is an open system who is exposed to environmental stressors, and thus requires lines of defense and reactions (Neuman, 1972). The main role of the *nurse* in Neuman's theory is reduction of stressors and protection of the client.

Madeleine Leininger

A cultural anthropologist, Leininger developed a culture care theory based on her work with clients of different cultures. A nurse by background, she wanted to understand why clients from various cultures responded differently to nursing care. She describes *nursing* as a learned humanistic art that is concerned with caring. The recipients of nursing care are *clients*, who may be individuals, families, groups, communities, and institutions in diverse health systems. Each person is influenced by his or her *environment*, which is made up of the politics, religion(s), education, values, and beliefs of the respective culture (Leininger, 1978). *Health* is culturally defined, and varies according to societal beliefs and practices.

Rosemarie Parse

Parse's theory of human becoming is based on the belief that a person is a living unity who participates in health experiences. According to Parse, the *client* maintains an open, mutual, constant interchange with the *environment* (Parse

1981). *Health* is viewed by Parse as a lived experience that is a process of being and becoming for the client. *Nursing* is concerned with the health of clients as they relate to their environment, and is directed toward assisting clients to find meaning in health experiences.

Jean Watson

The central theme of Jean Watson's theory of nursing is caring. She established the Center for Human Caring at the University of Colorado, whose purpose is the study of human caring and healing as the basis for nursing practice. Watson has identified ten "carative factors" in her theory, which are a combination of nursing interventions. She views *nursing* as a caring science based on curative factors and illness prevention. A fully functional, integrated self, the *client* is the focus of human caring. *Health* and illness are based on harmony or disharmony, respectively, within the body, mind, and soul (Watson, 1985). The *environment* is composed of internal (mental and spiritual well-being) and external (safety and physical comfort) aspects.

Each of these theorists has described nursing from a different perspective. Although many theories of nursing have been proposed, none has truly captured the complex nature of nursing. According to Meleis (1997), a discipline that deals with human beings has a need for multiple theories to address all phenomena associated with the discipline. In actual nursing practice, it may be useful to utilize one theory for one particular client's care, and another for a different situation. Portions of two or more theories may be found in use with each client. The remainder of the chapter discusses the application of nursing theory to practice.

THE RELATIONSHIP OF NURSING THEORY TO PRACTICE AND RESEARCH

If nursing possesses a body of knowledge, what means are used by nursing theorists to identify that knowledge? We have said nursing scholars rely on personal experiences and education to supply data from which to hypothesize relationships between concepts. Are experiences based on personal interpretations credible enough to be considered common knowledge for all nurses? Do you feel comfortable adopting any one of the previously discussed theorists' works into your daily practice with no questions asked? Would you be more likely to accept a theory that is based on scientific principles established by research findings?

Carper (1978) identified four patterns of knowing in nursing: (1) empirical—the science of nursing, based on research; (2) aesthetic—the art of nursing, based on intuitively understanding what to do; (3) personal—interpersonal contacts, therapeutic relationships, and individualized client care; and (4) ethical—the moral component of nursing. These patterns suggest that nursing knowledge comes from both scientific research and personal interactions with clients. Perhaps, then, nursing knowledge is a combination of science, art, intuition, interpersonal interactions, and moral behavior (Figure 4–4).

However, in order for nursing to claim to be a profession, ongoing research is essential to generate knowledge and validate nursing theories. Originally, nursing research was based on the scientific method and patterned after research from the natural and physical sciences. With the emergence of nursing theories that emphasize humanistic approaches to client care (such as the work of Parse and Watson), nurse researchers have begun to examine human experiences and behavioral responses more closely. According to Meleis (1997), nursing is a human science; therefore, nursing research should reflect the human aspects of nursing.

To the majority of practicing nurses, research findings are rarely considered in daily client care. In a clinical setting, nursing research is most often conducted by advanced practice nurses. However, practicing nurses play a major role in identifying researchable client problems and assisting to gather research data.

Research findings must be communicated to practicing nurses in order for nursing theory and research—important aspects of nursing care—to be fully understood and used to plan client care. As a registered nurse, you will need to stay abreast of current clinically based research findings; it will be important for you to read nursing journals, for example, and attend seminars, particularly those in your specialty area.

Nursing theory, research, and practice are interrelated, as shown in Figure 4–5. Nurses who understand this relationship are more likely to support theory-

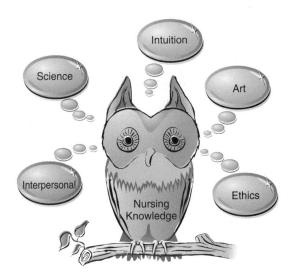

Figure 4–4
Nursing knowledge.

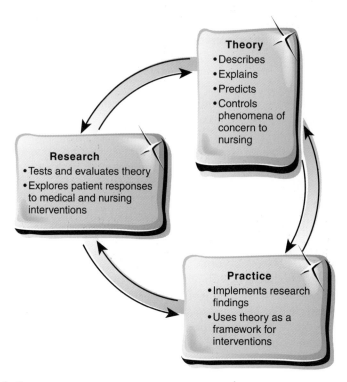

Figure 4–5
Relationship between nursing theory, research, and practice.

guided, research-based practice. This is essential in a health care environment that will continue to undergo significant changes in the twenty-first century (Walker and Redman, 1999).

How, you may be wondering, are you to relate nursing theory and research to your own nursing practice? In order to see the value of understanding the relationship, consider the following clinical scenario, which demonstrates the application of theory and research to nursing practice:

CLINICAL RESEARCH SCENARIO

Howard Miller, a 67-year-old retired steelworker, experienced a cerebro-vascular accident (CVA) one week ago. He has been admitted to a skilled nursing facility for rehabilitation care. Prior to the CVA, Howard was very active in church and community activities. His wife died four years ago, and he has been living three miles from his daughter and her family. The CVA has caused Howard to have difficulty speaking, swallowing, and moving his right arm and leg. In addition, he has developed skin breakdown over his coccyx. Howard has refused to participate in physical therapists' attempts to exercise his affected arm and leg, and will not assist nursing staff to reposition him in bed. He has told the occupational therapist that he wants to move in with his daughter's family so they may care for him.

Philip Sawyer, RN, has been assigned to be the primary nurse for Howard during his stay at the skilled nursing facility. Care planning will be a coordinated effort between Philip, Howard, his family, and other involved health care members. After completing an initial assessment on Howard, Philip formulates the following list of priority nursing diagnoses (see chapter 7):

1. Risk for aspiration related to depressed cough/gag reflexes
2. Impaired skin integrity related to effects of immobility as evidenced by ulcer on coccyx
3. Risk for infection related to altered integumentary system
4. Self-care deficit syndrome related to partial paralysis secondary to CVA as evidenced by inability to perform daily care activities

Philip believes many of Howard's problems stem from his self-care deficit, and plans to focus on developing outcomes and interventions that will encourage Howard to take a more active part in his care. He remembers studying about Dorothea Orem's self-care nursing theory, and recognizes that portions may help in planning care for Howard.

Recently, Philip attended a nursing seminar where he learned about new ways to motivate clients to participate in self-care. He heard a presenter share research findings from a study based on Orem's self-care theory. Using rehabilitation clients as subjects, the researcher examined how successful selected nursing interventions were at promoting self-care activities in the clients. Philip is eager to start applying some of the more successful strategies to Howard's care plan.

The nurse in this scenario uses Maslow's theory to prioritize nursing diagnoses and Orem's theory as a basis for understanding the client's responses to his illness. He recognizes the importance of theory-guided, research-based nursing practice.

Many nurses find it difficult to see the relevance of nursing theory and research to clinical practice, as evidenced by Suzanna's remarks in the opening scenario of the chapter. Much work remains to be done in bringing theory and research to the clinical arena, which should be the testing ground for both. The client's bedside should be the place for generating questions for research and testing theoretical assumptions.

How many times have you questioned why nurses perform a skill a particular way? Do you know if there is research to support the principles behind the procedure? It is the responsibility of every nurse to practice in a manner that supports the knowledge base of our profession. This can be accomplished only by recognizing the linkages among theory, research, and practice in nursing.

CRITICAL THINKING EXERCISES

1. Besides the four common concepts found in most nursing theories, make a personal list of concepts that you believe are important to the body of nursing knowledge:

    _____

    _____

    _____

    _____

    _____

    _____

2. Discuss the application of Hans Selye's stress/adaptation theory to the care of a postoperative client:

    _____

    _____

    _____

    _____

    _____

    _____

3. Using Jean Watson's theory of human caring, develop a client care plan for a young adult who has been diagnosed with ulcerative colitis.

    _____

    _____

    _____

    _____

    _____

4. Based on the care plan from question 3, discuss how you would go about ensuring that your care is research-based.

    _____

    _____

    _____

_____

_____

_____

REFERENCES

American Nurses' Association (1995). *Nursing: A social policy statement.* Washington, D.C.

Carper, B. (1978). Fundamental patterns of knowing in nursing. *Advances in Nursing Science* 1(1):13–23.

Catalano, J. (1996). *Contemporary professional nursing.* Philadelphia: F.A. Davis.

Craven, R., and C. Hirnle (2000). *Fundamentals of nursing: Human health and function* (3rd ed.). Philadelphia: Lippincott Williams & Wilkins.

Erikson, E. (1950). *Childhood and society* (2nd ed.). New York: Norton.

Leininger, M. (1978). *Transcultural nursing: Concepts, theories, and practices.* New York: John Wiley & Sons.

Maslow, A. (1954). *Motivation and personality.* New York: Harper & Row.

Massey, V. (1998). Theories and models of nursing practice. In *Foundations of nursing practice: A nursing process approach,* J. Leahy and P. Kizilay, eds. Philadelphia: W.B. Saunders.

Meleis, A. (1997). *Theoretical nursing: Development and progress* (3rd ed.). Philadelphia: Lippincott-Raven.

Neuman, B. (1972). *The Neuman systems model: Application to nursing education and practice.* New York: Appleton-Century-Crofts.

Nightingale, F. (1860). *Notes on nursing: What it is and what it is not.* London: Harrison & Sons.

Orem, D. (1971). *Nursing: Concepts of practice* (3rd ed.). New York: McGraw-Hill.

Parse, R. (1981). *Man-living-health: Theory of nursing.* New York: John Wiley & Sons.

Peplau, H. (1952). *Interpersonal relations in nursing.* New York: Putnam.

Rogers, M. (1986). Science of unitary human beings. In *Explorations on Martha Rogers' science of unitary human beings,* V. Malinski, ed. Norwalk, CT: Appleton-Century-Crofts.

Rolfe, G. (1996). *Closing the theory–practice gap.* Oxford, England: Butterworth-Heinemann.

Roy, C., and H. Andrews (1991). *The Roy adaptation model: The definitive statement.* Norwalk, CT: Appleton and Lange.

Selye, H. (1950). *The physiology and pathology of exposure to stress: A treatise based on the concepts of general adaptation syndrome and the disease of adaptation.* Montreal: Acta.

Upton, D. (1999). How can we achieve evidence-based practice if we have a theory–practice gap in nursing today? *Journal of Advanced Nursing* 29(3):549–555.

von Bertalanffy, L. (1968). *General systems theory: Foundations, development, applications.* New York: George Braziller.

Walker, P., and R. Redman (1999). Theory-guided, evidence-based reflective practice. *Nursing Science Quarterly* 12(4):298–303.

Watson, J. (1985). *Nursing: Human science and human care.* Norwalk, CT: Appleton-Century-Crofts.

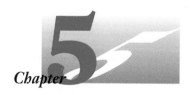

Chapter

Communicating Effectively

LEARNING OBJECTIVES

After completing this chapter, you will be able to:

1. Use effective communication techniques in a variety of settings.
2. Discuss specific nursing interventions that foster a therapeutic nurse–client relationship.
3. Identify strategies to improve communication with children.
4. Discuss age-related physical and cognitive changes that can affect communication with the elderly.
5. Apply effective communication techniques to care of clients and families in crisis.
6. Identify communication strategies that encourage a positive working relationship among nurses and other health care professionals.

Communication
Networking

Nonverbal
Communication

Therapeutic
Communication

 Maria, Kevin, and Suzanna are talking together in the hallway outside the classroom prior to a nursing exam.

Suzanna: Maria, you look pretty upset. Has something happened since we all studied together last night?

Maria: Yes, my husband and I had a fight after I got home. He thinks I'm spending too much time away from the family. He says he understands that I have to study a great deal for these tests, but he still resents the time I'm away from home. Before I even knew what was happening, our discussion turned into a major disagreement.

Kevin: Boy, the last thing you need right now is conflict! We're stressed enough as it is. Try to relax for now and concentrate on the test. Afterwards, we'll get together again. Maybe we can help you work through how to talk things out with him. Sometimes people don't communicate in a very positive manner, especially when they're upset.

As nurses, we interact with clients, families, communities, and other health care workers. We communicate through a variety of media—written charts, spoken language, telephones, fax machines, and computers. Effective communication allows us to establish harmonious, positive working relationships. Ineffective communication, on the other hand, can create tension and mistrust.

The nurse must establish therapeutic relationships with clients and families so that mutual trust and respect are evident. As a health care team leader, the registered nurse must be able to coordinate care, network with others, and collaborate on health care problems. Effective communication with other health care professionals is essential to the continuity of quality client care.

Because of expanded roles for nurses in today's changing health care environment, a more complex set of communication skills is required than was needed in previous years (Arnold and Boggs, 1999). Nurses must be able to converse with people from all walks of life, and in all settings. Consumers demand more information about available options

in health care, and nurses are in a strategic position to provide meaningful answers.

During your practical/vocational nursing program, you probably discussed
communication theory and guidelines for effective communication. At the registered nurse level, however, you will be called upon to exercise refined communication skills when participating in care planning, delegating to others, and resolving problems. The purpose of this chapter is to provide LPN/LVN to RN
bridge students with a better understanding of the nature of communication in
nursing. Basic communication techniques will be discussed, followed by application to the therapeutic nurse–client relationship. Communication strategies for
various age groups and clients and families will be explored, as well as suggestions
for improving communication among members of the health care team.

INTERPERSONAL COMMUNICATION

Communication may be defined as the process of imparting information, exchanging ideas, and expressing one's self in such a way as to be understood
(Gerace, 2000). All communication consists of three components—a message,
a sender, and a receiver. Communication between individuals may be either
one-way or two-way (Figure 5–1). During one-way communication, one person
dominates the conversation, and little, if any, feedback is given from the second
person. Two-way communication involves mutual sharing of information with
the chance for each to provide feedback and engage in a dynamic exchange
(Sieh and Brentin, 1997). It therefore stands to reason that nurses need to be
aware of the effectiveness of two-way communication in order to provide clients,
families, and other professionals the opportunity to participate in care planning.

The message being sent is not always perceived as intended; therefore, two-
way communication, which allows for clarification and questions, is a more
effective form of communication (Sieh and Brentin, 1997). Factors such as past
experiences, cultural differences, the environment, body language, and tone of
voice can affect how the message is perceived. A sender's verbal message may
have one meaning, while nonverbal cues such as posture and facial expression
actually convey another. Consider the following scenario:

> Misty is a new graduate nurse who is caring for Bryan, a 23-year-old man
> who has had surgery to repair a shoulder injury. Bryan has requested extra
> portions of food on his dinner tray, but has received a normal-sized meal
> from the dietary department for the past two evenings. When Bryan summons
> Misty to his room to complain, she is extremely busy with another client,
> and resents being interrupted to deal with what she regards as a minor
> concern. Upon entering Bryan's room, Misty displays tense body lan-
> guage—her arms are crossed over her chest and her face is set in firm
> lines. As Bryan expresses his complaint, Misty begins to tap one foot and

sigh loudly. She tells Bryan in a curt voice that she will be very happy to call for extra food portions for him, spins quickly around, and leaves the room before he can say another word.

If you were Bryan, how would you feel? Would you believe that Misty was happy to try to obtain extra food for you? All too often, nurses convey a negative form of communication to clients who are attempting to express needs. Misty may have actually called the dietary department for Bryan's food, but she

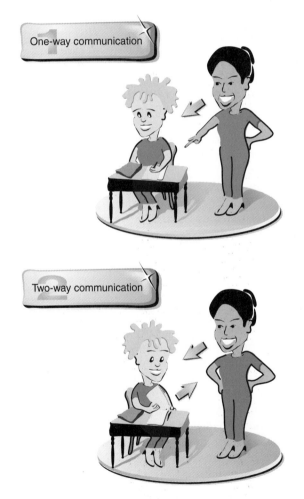

Figure 5-1
Components of communication.

certainly did not give him reason to believe she was doing so out of concern for his well-being.

Nonverbal communication may actually speak more loudly than verbal communication, as in the above example (Sieh and Brentin, 1997). Examples of nonverbal cues include:

- posture (tense, relaxed, aggressive, hostile, friendly)
- use of eye contact (looks at other person, avoids eye contact)
- tone of voice (agitated, angry, caring, concerned)
- proximity of message sender to receiver (near, distant)
- use of gestures (waving arms, clenched fists, arms relaxed)

When nonverbal communication is inconsistent with what is expressed verbally, the message receiver can be confused as to the intended meaning. People are usually very responsive to nonverbal cues, so care must be taken to avoid conveying contradictory information.

Interpersonal communication may be enhanced by behaviors that convey a sense of respect, concern, and interest. Following is a list of suggested behaviors that encourage more effective communication with clients and others:

1. Sit or stand with your body directly facing the other person in order to give the impression of being completely tuned in to communicating with him/her.
2. Unless culturally inappropriate, make eye contact while talking as well as listening in order to give the other person your full attention.
3. Assume a relaxed body posture; let your arms rest straight at your sides and fold your hands in your lap if you are sitting. Legs should be still and relaxed.
4. Ask for clarification of information when needed. Do not assume you can determine what the other person means if you are unsure.
5. Use silence appropriately. Allow the other person to communicate what is important to him/her. Do not dominate the conversation. Practice listening more than talking.
6. Treat the other person respectfully and in a caring manner. Attempt to convey a genuine interest in and concern for his or her needs. When appropriate, touch the client gently when comfort is needed.
7. If at all possible, do not give the impression of needing to be somewhere else at that moment. Try to make the other person feel as if you have time for him/her and that his/her needs are important to you.
8. Provide information to the client/family when needed so that informed decisions can be made about care. When information changes, be sure to keep the client updated.
9. Ask open-ended questions in order to encourage clients to answer and communicate information. One-word responses reveal very little about clients' feelings.

10. Acknowledge that you hear what the client is saying. Do not interrupt clients abruptly. Allow them to describe their concerns and needs completely.

It is important for nurses to remember that a caring, interested attitude encourages clients to feel more at ease and trusting of health care professionals. As a result, there is a greater likelihood of a positive outcome in the communication process.

COMMUNICATION WITH CLIENTS

Hildegard Peplau, a nursing theorist (chapter 4), describes **therapeutic communication** between the nurse and client as central in providing effective nursing care (Peplau, 1997). She believes this unique form of communication between the nurse and client fosters respect and self-worth. According to Peplau, an effective nurse–client relationship will:

- enhance client well-being
- promote recovery
- encourage client self-care

A "helping" relationship, such as that between a nurse and client, involves taking the responsibility for helping one who is seeking help (Arnold and Boggs, 1999). In this relationship, the nurse must focus intently on becoming aware of the client's feelings and needs. This involves entering into the private world of the client and participating in personal discussions that sometimes include confidential material.

Confidentiality often becomes an issue in nurse–client relationships when nurses are made privy to information of a sensitive nature (see chapter 10). When clients become comfortable enough to communicate personal information to nurses, they have the right to expect that the information will be used for health care purposes only. Nurses need to be aware of cultural differences, as some groups do not share private information as readily as others.

Personal prejudices and preformed opinions must be put aside in order to listen openly to what clients are expressing (Figure 5–2). Some clients have personal value systems that differ greatly from those of the nurses who care for them. Consider the following scenario:

> Eric is an emergency department nurse who has been assigned to care for a gang member who participated in a drive-by shooting in which a five-year-old boy was hit by gunfire. The gang member was shot accidentally in the knee and has been calling for pain medication since arriving in the emergency department. Eric has been informed that the five-year-old boy has died.

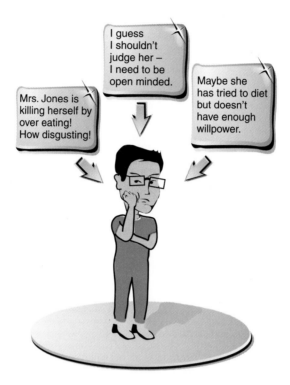

Figure 5–2
Put aside personal prejudices.

In emotional situations such as this, nurses often have difficulty entering into a caring, concerned relationship with a client. If you were Eric, would you have to identify and set aside personal prejudices regarding the client before you could care for him?

Describe the steps you would take to prepare yourself to provide nonjudgmental care for this client:

_____

_____

_____

_____

_____

_____

As nurses, we must develop skills that allow us to respond to clients effectively, regardless of the challenges involved. Practice using the previously suggested behaviors that encourage positive communication, such as listening attentively, making eye contact, responding in a respectful manner, and assuming a relaxed stance. The groundwork for a continuing therapeutic nurse–client relationship may be laid by simply meeting a client's immediate needs in a caring manner.

Establishing a comfortable method of communicating with clients also involves the way in which we address them. Upon meeting a client, introduce yourself and give your full title. You should also inform the client about your role in his or her care. Unless clients ask to be called by their first name, address them as Mr., Mrs., Miss, Ms., and so forth, followed by their last name unless you are caring for a child. This establishes a professional relationship between the nurse and the client and sets the boundaries of the therapeutic relationship. Avoid the use of terms such as "honey," "sweetie," "baby," and the like when addressing clients. Such labels belittle clients and are examples of unprofessional behavior (Sieh and Brentin, 1997).

Communicating effectively requires time, energy, and the ability to focus on what the other person is attempting to convey. Various factors may affect a client's ability to communicate effectively:

- illness
- stress
- sleep deprivation
- sedation
- language barriers
- cognitive dysfunction
- cultural differences
- mistrust
- the environment

Nurses must assess clients and families for potential barriers to communication and develop interventions accordingly. For example, a client in pain may also be sleep-deprived; therefore, effective communication could be hampered by the client's inability to focus. The nurse could plan to medicate the client and allow time for sleep before communicating important information. Clients' family members and close friends can also be utilized for communication purposes. Language barriers and cultural differences may be overcome by involving clients' relatives to translate information and explain personal preferences. Limited privacy, an uncomfortable environment, and noise may also interfere with the nurse's ability to communicate effectively with the client. Nurses should always be mindful of providing privacy for clients when communicating personal information.

Finally, during therapeutic communication, nurses must respect clients' personal space, or the invisible emotional boundary needed for interpersonal com-

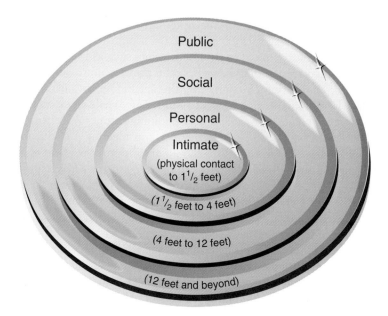

Figure 5–3
Personal space boundaries.

fort (Arnold and Boggs, 1999). As shown in Figure 5–3, humans allow others within differing proximities of themselves, depending on the level of familiarity (Hall, 1969). An initial assessment of the client will reveal cultural and developmental factors that affect personal space boundaries. For example, males of certain cultures are not at ease having nonfamily members touch them in a comforting manner. Communicating with clients should always be centered around creating an environment of mutual respect and trust.

DEVELOPMENTAL CONSIDERATIONS

Because of developmental differences, communication strategies used with adults may not be effective with infants, children, and older adults. Many nurses report that they feel more comfortable talking with clients of their own age group, for they have more in common. It is, however, important to understand similarities and differences when communicating with people of all ages.

When caring for a child, both the child and parents are clients. In other words, nurses must remember to develop a positive relationship with both. The parents or guardians contribute a great deal of information about the child, especially if the child is very young and unable to communicate clearly. When communicating with a child, the nurse must adapt the message to the developmental level of the child (Wong, 1999). Box 5–1 contains suggested communication tips for various age groups of children.

Honesty is an essential component of any form of communication with a child. Because of the concrete nature of their thinking patterns, children respond in a more positive manner if told the truth consistently. It is imperative that nurses develop a trusting relationship with child clients if expected outcomes are to be met.

Nurses should also remember that young children tend to take what is said literally. For example, a child who is told an injection will be "a little stick" may actually believe that a part of a tree will be used!

Box 5-1   *Communication with Children*

Infants

- Involve parents as much as possible
- Hold, rock, and cuddle to reassure
- Use a soothing tone of voice
- Get at child's eye level

Toddlers

- Use simple sentences
- Allow some autonomy
- Show interest in the child's toys
- Be honest about painful procedures

Preschoolers

- Focus on the present, not what will happen later
- Use play therapy to explain procedures
- Offer some choices
- Use concrete explanations

School Age

- Explain illness and procedures in simple terms
- Allow children to assist with their own care
- Respect privacy when a child is changing or bathing
- Play age-appropriate games with the child

Adolescents

- Allow teenagers to participate in decision making
- Provide privacy
- Be available to listen without being judgmental
- Expect and accept regressive behavior

There is no magic age at which adults become known as "older adults"; however, the beginning of the latter stage of the life cycle is frequently cited as 65 (Arnold and Boggs, 1999). Because of the commonly accepted stereotype of the elderly client who cannot see or hear well, many nurses assume these clients are also less mentally competent. Some elderly clients do indeed have diminished mental capacities and have difficulty performing self-care. That does not, however, render them incapable of communication. Nurses should become familiar with age-related changes in the elderly that interfere with effective communication patterns so care planning may be adjusted to meet their special needs. Some of the factors that affect communication with the elderly are:

- visual, auditory, tactile deficits
- fatigue
- illness
- anxiety
- depression
- confusion
- fear
- loneliness
- altered sleep patterns
- medication side effects

Many of the physical changes that occur with aging can affect the client's overall sense of well-being and self-esteem (Ebersole and Hess, 1998). The elderly frequently experience loneliness and depression after losing a spouse and, upon entering a health care system, may demonstrate dependent behavior. Upon initial assessment of an elderly client, it is essential for the nurse to gather pertinent physical and psychosocial data that will influence future communication.

Regardless of the age of the client, the most important communication strategies are those aimed at honesty, mutual respect, and developing a sense of trust. Even though school-age children are too young to understand the details of illness, they still enjoy being directly addressed by health care professionals when information is being given to their parents. Older adults appreciate being advised of health care options, even if they require assistance from family members with decision making.

COMMUNICATION DURING CRISIS

In the process of caring for clients, you will witness a variety of emotional situations that range from the despair of an unwelcome diagnosis to the ecstasy of birth. As a registered nurse, you must be adaptable enough in your communication skills to support clients through these challenges.

During times of change, people experience varying degrees of stress, which may bring about alterations in behavior. A sudden disruption in life's plans can strain coping abilities of clients and their families. Consider the following scenario:

> Cindy is a 31-year-old who has just been informed that she has cancer of the uterus and must have a hysterectomy. She has been married six months, and she and her husband have been planning to start a family in about a year. Shawn, Cindy's nurse on the surgical unit, stopped in her room to change the IV solution and found her crying uncontrollably. Cindy admitted to Shawn that she and her husband had just had an argument over her inability to have the children they had planned.

How should Shawn handle this situation? What would be the most effective way to communicate with Cindy?

_____

_____

_____

_____

_____

_____

How would *you* address the needs of Cindy's husband?

_____

_____

_____

_____

_____

_____

As nurses, we are called upon to soothe both physical and emotional wounds. Despite busy daily routines, nurses may have to stop to tend to a dying client's loved ones or assist a physician with informing a client of a poor prognosis. Few professionals experience the range of emotional responses from clients that nurses do. You, the nurse, can help clients through life's crises by allowing them to feel comfortable enough to talk with you and express their needs. Families can be assisted to develop meaningful ways to communicate with loved ones by effective use of the therapeutic relationship (Leske, 1998).

Few crises are as trying in life as that associated with the imminent death of a loved one. Nurses must be able to identify and understand reactions from clients and families when they are experiencing grief. Box 5–2 lists nursing interventions that focus on assisting grieving clients and families.

People deal with grief in a variety of ways; some adapt in a healthy way, while others do not. From the initial shock and disbelief associated with unplanned death to final acceptance and healthy bereavement, people use a multitude of coping mechanisms to handle the stress. Some of the more common emotions are denial, disbelief, anger, and fear. Since nurses spend more time with clients than other health care professionals, many of the behaviors that stem from these emotions are directed toward them. The following suggestions may help nurses deal with negative responses from clients/family members in a positive manner:

1. Remain calm—do not allow yourself to become angry and emotional in response to another person's behavior. Try to remember where the negative behavior is coming from and do not take it personally.
2. Speak slowly and carefully when confronted with anger. Repetition may be necessary, as agitated people have difficulty focusing on what is being said to them.
3. Do not intrude into the personal space of an angry person. Allow time for clients to calm down before performing nursing interventions that require close contact.
4. Discuss ways in which the client's concerns may be addressed. Try to emphasize things that are attainable, rather than dwelling on what cannot be changed.
5. Attempt to convey a caring, empathetic attitude. Explain to the client and family that you are there to help them in any way you can.
6. Enlist the aid of crisis intervention teams or other resource personnel that may be available to assist with negative forms of behavior.

Box 5–2 *Nursing Interventions for Grieving Clients and Families*

- Assist clients to verbalize their feelings
- Explain procedures and treatments
- Help clients to attain or maintain optimal health
- Encourage clients to surround themselves with favorite belongings
- Assist families with coping strategies
- Provide information about needed resources
- Maximize comfort, minimize stress
- Encourage the development of support systems
- Assist to find meaning in life and death

It is essential to understand that clients and families need your assistance during times of stress, regardless of the type of behavior they exhibit. Even if you expect anger to be directed toward you, be available to listen to concerns from clients. By displaying an attitude that shows you are interested in the client's welfare, you are more likely to be of greater help (Czerwiec, 1996). Involve family members in discussions when information is being provided in order to strengthen family support systems. Help families to mobilize resources and participate in decision making, as they may feel helpless and overwhelmed when grieving (Arnold and Boggs, 1999). By assisting families in crisis to set short-term, realistic goals, nurses can help them focus on the immediate future and begin to work toward a positive resolution.

COMMUNICATION WITH OTHER HEALTH CARE PROFESSIONALS

Nurses must be able to extend the positive communication skills utilized with clients and families to interactions with other members of the health care team. While planning and coordinating client care, nurses interact with a variety of other people, such as dietitians, respiratory therapists, pharmacists, and physicians. Smooth communication among health care workers enhances the delivery of care, whereas inadequate or negative interactions may actually cause client care to suffer (Chitty, 1997). Interdisciplinary care planning is becoming more essential as hospital stays shorten. Therefore, it is imperative for nurses to effectively communicate their portion of the care plan to the rest of the team.

Historically, nurses have taken a passive role with respect to the physician in client care planning. As gender role changes occur in society, it has become more accepted for women to have a greater voice in decision making. Because of the need to maximize client outcomes, nurses are taking a more active part in collaboration activities with physicians. Collaboration, by definition, involves interaction between individuals who share knowledge and expertise to meet a common goal (Stichler, 1995). This allows for greater information sharing, and in the case of clients, a more comprehensive plan of care (Arnold and Boggs, 1999). Nurses collaborate with many other professionals in regard to client care, such as religious counselors, physical therapists, social workers, and other nurses.

Increased autonomy and input into decision making brings more opportunity for interpersonal conflict between nurses and other health care professionals (see Chapter 9 for a discussion on conflict management). The following suggestions may help prevent negative communication with others:

1. Listen to the opinions and ideas of others. Do not interrupt to impose your views into the conversation. Wait until it is your turn.
2. Treat other members of the team with respect: Their suggestions are important.

3. Practice assertive, rather than aggressive, behavior. State your ideas clearly and competently without attacking those of others.
4. Be flexible. It may be necessary to bend or reject your suggestions in order to design the best care plan for the client.
5. Accept criticism with an open mind. Try to be objective about why your suggestions are not acceptable to others and learn from the experience. Do not view criticism as a personal attack.
6. Do not respond to others with anger. To do so causes further anger and interferes with the ability to work together harmoniously.

These tips may sound like good recommendations, but what if you are on the receiving end of a co-worker's anger or unpleasant behavior (Figure 5–4)?

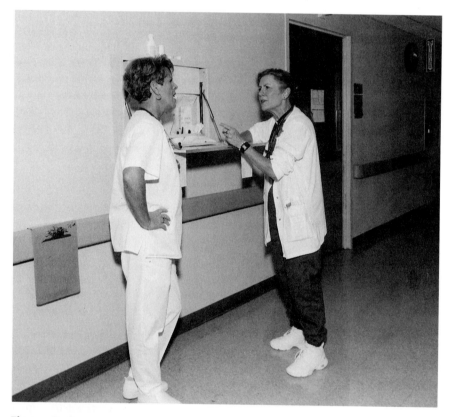

Figure 5–4
Interpersonal communication may result in conflict.

If this happens, try to respond without becoming emotional. Investigate the cause of his/her behavior and take steps to deal with the situation in an assertive manner (Sallee, 1999). The following suggestions may help you to handle negative verbal behavior from a colleague:

- Avoid responding in anger.
- Do not argue in front of others.
- Use an assertive, calm manner of speaking.
- State your position, listen to what the other person has to say.
- Provide an explanation for your actions, not excuses.
- Use relaxed, open body language.
- Do not act intimidated.
- Whether or not you resolve the disagreement, find a workable solution that is in the best interest of all the involved parties.

One method of improving communication among peers is networking. This involves sharing ideas and knowledge with other members of our profession. By communicating valuable information with others, nurses develop important resources. Networking allows us to build professional relationships within our own organizations, as well as with peers from great distances. Exposure to other ways of thinking improves our ability to problem solve and opens our minds to other possibilities. This exchange of information allows us to see the value of good communication skills.

Communication with colleagues takes place in other ways besides face-to-face encounters. Documentation of care has traditionally been on written nurses' notes and care plans. Recently, many health care organizations have computerized client records so that very little writing takes place, if any. Many systems allow nurses to access client data, obtain laboratory results, and create individualized care plans electronically. Nurses are recognizing the importance of computers as an aid to performing timely tasks.

Effective communication between nurses, clients, and other members of the health care team is essential to quality of care and achievement of client outcomes. As you enter the world of the registered nurse, you will be expected to employ communication strategies to deal with a variety of everyday problems. Whether you are providing comfort to the family of a dying client or delegating duties to assistive nursing personnel, the manner in which you communicate will determine how effective you are as a nurse. Problems will be brought to you, as a team leader, for resolution. By using effective therapeutic communication skills, you will be enhancing client care and growing as a professional.

CRITICAL THINKING EXERCISES

1. You and an aide are caring for an elderly woman in an extended care facility. As you assist the client to a chair in her room in order to clean her and the bed of incontinent feces, the daughter arrives and says, "This is disgusting! As much as we pay for the care of my mother here, the least you nurses could do is keep her clean." Discuss the feelings this sort of remark creates in you. What strategies could you use to deal effectively with negative communication?

_____

_____

_____

_____

_____

2. You have been assigned to care for a five-year-old girl with appendicitis. Describe nursing interventions aimed at fostering positive communication with the child based on her developmental level.

_____

_____

_____

_____

_____

3. Discuss communication techniques that could be used in caring for an 86-year-old man who is hospitalized with pneumonia. He has difficulty hearing, is widowed, and lives alone.

_____

_____

_____

_____

_____

_____

4. Consider ways in which you might develop a network of peers. Formulate a plan to begin actively networking with classmates in your LPN/LVN to RN transition program. What are some benefits you hope to reap?

_____

_____

_____

_____

_____

_____

REFERENCES

Arnold, E., and K. Boggs (1999). *Interpersonal relationships: Professional communication skills for nurses* (3rd ed.). Philadelphia: W.B. Saunders.

Chitty, K. (2001). Communication and collaboration in nursing. In *Professional nursing: Concepts and challenges* (3rd ed.), K. Chitty, ed. Philadelphia: W.B. Saunders.

Czerwiec, M. (1996). When a loved one is dying: Families talk about nursing care. *American Journal of Nursing* 96(5):32–36.

Ebersole, P., and P. Hess (1998). *Toward healthy aging: Human needs and nursing response* (5th ed.). St. Louis: C.V. Mosby.

Gerace, L. (2000). Communication: The nurse–client relationship. In *Fundamentals of nursing* (3rd ed.), R. Craven and C. Hirnle, eds. Philadelphia: Lippincott Williams & Wilkins.

Hall, E. (1969). *The hidden dimension.* Garden City, NJ: Doubleday.

Leske, J. (1998). Treatment for family members in crisis after critical injury. *AACN Clinical Issues* 9(1):129–139.

Peplau, H. (1997). Peplau's theory of interpersonal relations. *Nursing Science Quarterly* 10(4):162–167.

Sallee, A. (1999). Effective communication. In *Contemporary nursing: Issues, trends, and management,* B. Cherry and S. Jacob, eds. Philadelphia: C.V. Mosby.

Sieh, A., and L. Brentin (1997). *The nurse communicates. . . .* Philadelphia: W.B. Saunders.

Stichler, J. (1995). Professional interdependence: The art of collaboration. *Advanced Practice Nursing Quarterly* 1(1):53–61.

Wong, D., M. Hockenberry-Eaton, D. Wilson, M. Winkelstein, E. Ahmann, and P. DiVito-Thomas (1999). *Whaley and Wong's nursing care of infants and children* (6th ed.). Philadelphia: C.V. Mosby.

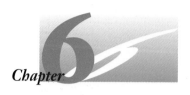

Thinking Skills
for the Registered Nurse

LEARNING OBJECTIVES

After completing this chapter, you will be able to:

1. Describe the importance of effective thinking skills to registered nursing practice.
2. Discuss the differences in traditional and higher level thinking.
3. Compare and contrast critical thinking, creative thinking, problem solving, and decision making.
4. Apply the use of thinking skills in planning nursing care for clients in various health care settings.

Creative Thinking	Decision Making	Problem Solving
Critical Thinking	Metacognition	Thinking Skills

 Maria, Kevin, and Suzanna are riding home together after the first three days of the LPN to RN bridge program. They are having a discussion of role differences of LPN/LVNs and RNs.

Suzanna: I really don't understand what all the confusion is about. This program just seems like a continuation of my practical nurse program.

Maria: Oh, I'd say my job as an LPN has been a lot like the job RNs do . . . at least the ones I work with. But, they always have to deal with problems that come up. I've been happy to avoid the hard decisions they have to be make. How about you, Kevin?

Kevin: I agree. I frequently help solve problems that occur at work, but I'm relieved to have an RN in charge—someone who's ultimately responsible for deciding what to do. That leaves me curious though. I really want to learn more about how you make big decisions. How do you know what the best course of action is when clients develop sudden problems?

Did you know that nurses can practice using thinking skills in much the same way they practice physical assessment, venipuncture, medication administration, and other psychomotor skills? Technical skills are important in nursing; but to survive in today's challenging health care climate, registered nurses also need the ability to think in a rational, analytical manner (Jacobs et al., 1997). As client care becomes more complex, the use of higher level thinking skills becomes essential.

This chapter is intended to help you understand the importance of using effective thinking processes when planning client care. After reading this chapter, you will be able to identify and refine your current methods of thinking, and thus become a higher level thinker. As you develop new ways of looking at the world of nursing, it is crucial that you recognize the change in mindset that accompanies your change in role. In order to think differently, your mind must be stretched to new dimensions so you are capable of processing information and dealing with it in a different manner.

As an RN you will be expected to think critically, problem solve, make decisions, and use creative thinking to formulate approaches to client care. You may find new ways to use old ways of thinking, for what you know now is only part of what you will know later. A change in thinking skills will bring new insights into nursing care, so allow yourself to welcome this change as one that will enrich your practice of nursing.

WHAT ARE THINKING SKILLS?

Thinking is a dynamic process—one that is constantly changing—and it is important for us to understand how we think in order to improve our thinking (Rubenfeld and Scheffer, 1995). All of us have developed our own individual thinking patterns, much as we have developed other personality characteristics. You may, for example, rely on memorization and total recall when asked a question, or you may prefer to analyze information before responding. Other commonly used methods of thinking are reasoning, relating, and reflecting (Swartz and Perkins, 1990).

If we have already developed a personal thinking style, how can we change it? Educational research has shown that new thinking skills may be learned and are enhanced by practice, eventually leading to a restructuring of thinking processes. This mental restructuring is important in the transition from LPN/ LVN to RN.

For our purposes in nursing, critical thinking, creative thinking, problem solving, and decision making are examples of thinking skills (Box 6–1). These are skills that are clearly important in everyday client care. So why is it important for us to discuss practicing these skills? Don't we already know how to solve problems and make decisions? Can we really say we are as competent as we could be when it comes to analyzing client problems and using good judgment?

A look at the benefits of good thinking might help you to see the importance of thinking skills in nursing. According to Swartz and Perkins (1990), better thinking yields:

- keener critical assessments
- more creative strategies
- deeper insights
- more reliable conclusions
- sounder decisions
- better end products

It would seem obvious that a nurse who improves her thinking in these ways is more efficient in planning client care. So how do we learn to use thinking skills? First we must be willing to analyze our current thought patterns, a process known as metacognition, or thinking about how we think. Then we must begin

Box 6-1   *Thinking Skills*

- Critical thinking
- Creative thinking
- Problem solving
- Decision making

to focus on practicing higher level thinking by applying thinking skills to everyday practice. Before learning to use each specific thinking skill, perhaps we need to examine the differences between traditional ways of thinking and higher level thinking.

TRADITIONAL VS. HIGHER LEVEL THINKING

Consider all the things you think about in a day's time, from the moment you wake up until you fall asleep. How many of these thoughts receive serious consideration? Do you carefully deliberate upon what to eat for breakfast? Or do you merely pull the same box of cereal from the cupboard without giving it much thought? Chances are, your breakfast choice is a habit, a mechanical repetition of previous actions. And it is much easier—and far more efficient—to repeat previous behavior than to stop and think through various alternatives every time you do something.

Certain decisions, however, are not habitual and clearly require more than brief consideration. You do not, for example, choose a new car unthinkingly nor decide to get married without contemplation. Such is the nature of health care, where each decision can seriously affect a client's ability to achieve optimum health.

All too often, nurses find themselves in a "rut"; they become used to providing the same type of interventions for clients with similar problems. When actions become routine, decisions are frequently made without taking the time to deliberate carefully and arrive at the best solution. Registered nurses must be able to determine when traditional forms of thinking should be replaced with higher level thinking when faced with client care decisions.

How can you distinguish between traditional thinking and higher level thinking? Lipman (1988) differentiates "ordinary thinking" from critical thinking, as shown in Table 6–1. From this comparison we can see that ordinary thinking relies heavily upon personal beliefs and judgments that may not be supported by facts. Higher level thinking, on the other hand, allows for more analysis of facts, broader thinking, and abstractions. In order to be effective nurses, we

TABLE 6-1
Comparison of Ordinary and Higher Level Thinking

ORDINARY THINKING	HIGHER LEVEL THINKING
Guessing	Estimating
Preferring	Evaluating
Grouping	Classifying
Believing	Assuming
Inferring	Inferring logically
Associating concepts	Grasping principles
Noting relationships	Noting relationships among other relationships
Supposing	Hypothesizing
Offering opinions without reasons	Offering opinions with reasons
Making judgments without criteria	Making judgments with criteria

From Lipman, M. (1988). Critical thinking—What can it be? *Educational Leadership* 46:38–43, with permission from ASCD. All rights reserved.

must be able to look past previous suppositions and form opinions based on analysis of data. Read the following scenario and possible outcomes, then answer the related question:

> Mary Gatewood, the night nurse on a busy surgical nursing unit, is called to the room of Mr. Foster, an 87-year-old who had a colon resection two days ago. He is crying and tells Mary that he "hurts so much" and "needs something to sleep."
>
> > *Outcome One:* Mary checks his orders and finds that he may have medication for pain as needed. After giving him a narcotic injection, Mary turns out the light, closes his door, and returns to her other responsibilities.
> >
> > *Outcome Two:* Mary questions him further regarding his specific problem and determines that his back is hurting from lying in one position for several hours. She checks his vital signs, assesses his surgical incision for signs of bleeding, redness, or other abnormality, and asks if he has any abdominal pain. When he denies any other difficulty besides an aching back, Mary repositions Mr. Foster, rubs his back, and encourages deep-breathing exercises to help him relax. As he dozes off to sleep, Mary returns to her other responsibilities.

Which of these two outcomes demonstrates the use of ordinary thinking and which demonstrates higher level thinking? Why?

_____

_____

_____

_____

_____

_____

How many times do situations similar to the first outcome actually occur in nursing practice? Shouldn't we, as nurses, be committed to providing the most effective and efficient care possible to our clients? This can be accomplished if we learn the use of thinking skills to assist us in our daily lives. What are some of the benefits of learning to use better thinking skills? You will begin to:

- view problems as challenges
- become tolerant of ambiguity
- consider more alternatives
- become more self-critical
- become more open-minded
- use persistence to problem solve
- search for evidence
- revise goals when necessary

In general, the higher level thinker has the ability to analyze problems and arrive at rational decisions more effectively than the ordinary thinker.

Let's now take a close look at four specific thinking skills: critical thinking, creative thinking, problem solving, and decision making. You'll find that these skills are similar in many ways, and that they are very important tools in planning nursing care for clients and families. As illustrated in Figure 6–1, creative thinking, problem solving, and decision making are components of critical thinking, which is more broadly defined (see the following discussion).

CRITICAL THINKING

As discussed previously, thinking may be aimless and mechanical, or it may be controlled, purposeful, and analytical. Critical thinking is an example of "reasonable, reflective thinking that is focused on deciding what to believe or do" (Ennis, 1987). It is a dynamic process, and has been defined by various

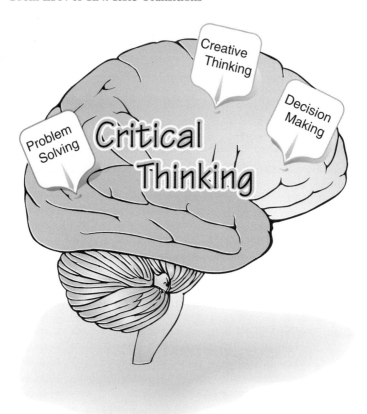

Figure 6-1
Thinking skills for nursing.

authors as "purposeful," "intellectually disciplined," and "logical." These descriptions probably sound rather vague, so let's discuss several qualities of critical thinkers in order to gain a better understanding of the skill.

A wealth of material has been written about critical thinking and what it means to be a critical thinker. The following is an overall description of the characteristics of the critical thinker.

The Critical Thinker:

- thinks on many levels, from simple memorization to higher level synthesis
- has the ability to solve problems using an organized approach
- has the ability to think independently of others
- is able to analyze arguments and distinguish fact from opinion

- seeks a clear understanding of the main question
- attempts to be well informed
- takes the entire situation into account
- is open-minded and fair
- seeks precision
- employs organized strategies of reasoning

So how, you may be asking yourself, do you learn to be a critical thinker? The answer lies in learning to analyze your own patterns of thinking, then in practicing the characteristics described above. For example, think of a recent situation in which you were required to make a decision regarding a problem of some sort. Answer the following questions:

What was the problem (in as much detail as you can remember)?

_____

_____

_____

_____

_____

_____

List the steps you took to solve the problem, including the rationale:

_____

_____

_____

_____

_____

Now ask yourself:

- Did I fully understand the problem?
- Did I gather all available data in order to look at the whole problem?
- Did I determine the validity of the data?
- Was I open-minded?
- Did I try my best to separate fact from opinion and emotion?
- Was my thinking approach organized and logical?
- Did I try to think for myself and not be swayed by popular opinion?

- Did I strive to be precise and make the most informed decision?
- Has my own personal point of view influenced my thinking?

This method of self-analysis will improve your awareness of your thought patterns, and will encourage more insight into critical thinking behaviors. Again, this method of thinking is a skill, and must be consciously practiced until it is unconsciously incorporated into daily life as habit.

How does this use of critical thinking apply to nursing? By virtue of the close contact that we have with our clients' personal lives, we have always been called upon to use reasoning abilities in choosing appropriate courses of action. In other words, critical thinking is nothing new in nursing. So why has critical thinking suddenly become a popular topic of discussion?

Health care is moving with increasing frequency into the community and home environments. This means that client care decisions will become more complex as nurses must function more independently. Therefore, registered nurses must be fully prepared to approach each situation with the logical and systematic approach used in critical thinking. Let's look at how we can specifically relate critical thinking to nursing.

Various nursing authors have attempted to define critical thinking as it applies to nursing. It has been described as thinking based on scientific principles: It is "reasonable and reflective" and "goal-directed," and it "aims to make judgments based on facts rather than guesswork" (Alfaro-LeFevre, 1999). Inherent in the thinking skill is the ability to problem solve creatively by using intuition. According to Allen (1997), critical thinkers determine priorities in client care and work with others to make decisions. From these definitions, it would seem that critical thinking in nursing is a skill that involves the following components (Figure 6–2):

- the ability to utilize a scientific knowledge base effectively
- the use of a systematic, logical approach to decision making
- a willingness to search for and evaluate all pertinent assessment data
- the ability to think independently and work cooperatively
- the appropriate use of nursing intuition

The registered nurse who strives to incorporate these characteristics into her way of thinking is one who does not accept things at face value, but continually searches for a deeper understanding of all aspects of a situation. In order to become this type of thinker, you must practice applying the components of a critical thinker to the nursing care you provide. For example, consider the following scenario:

> Ginger Lange, 17 years old, has been admitted to your nursing unit with a diagnosis of pyelonephritis. She has an order for antibiotics to be given three times a day. You are assigned to care for her on the day shift.

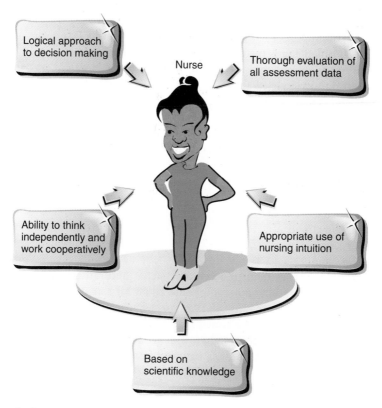

Figure 6-2
Critical thinking in nursing.

What information do you need to know before giving the medication to this client?

_____

_____

_____

_____

_____

_____

If you said that you would (1) ask the client about allergies, (2) make sure you are familiar with side effects of the drug, and (3) follow the five rights of medication administration, you are correct. However, as a critical thinker, there's more to do. You would also check the client's lab work to see if a urine culture and sensitivity supports the use of that particular antibiotic. If not, the physician should be notified for a medication change. In addition, you would want to assess the client's temperature, white blood cell count, amount of pain when voiding, and appetite level in order to evaluate how well the medication is working. Your client should also be assessed for knowledge of her illness and treatment program, and appropriate client teaching should be done.

You may be wondering by now if the process of critical thinking takes more time than ordinary thinking. In many health care facilities, it is not unusual for a nurse to be assigned to care for eight to ten acutely ill clients. Do nurses really have the time to gather data about problems, carefully analyze the information, and implement comprehensive client care? When practiced routinely, critical thinking replaces previous ways of approaching problems, and is actually no more time consuming. In fact, nurses who use logical, sound methods to make clinical decisions may prevent health complications, thereby reducing the length of illness in clients.

Far too often nurses tend to accept the status quo rather than develop the habit of thinking carefully and completely about all aspects of client care. By learning how to think more critically, you as a registered nurse will find yourself better prepared for future challenges in nursing. Don't be afraid to take the time to analyze data more thoroughly; you will find that in the long run client care outcomes will improve, nursing care will become more fulfilling, and your self-confidence will receive a welcome boost.

CREATIVE THINKING

How is creative thinking related to nursing practice? Is it a necessary part of a registered nurse's repertoire of skills? Consider the following scenario:

> Carla James is an RN who is making a home visit on Freda Carroll, an 86-year-old who has chronic heart failure. Mrs. Carroll takes digoxin and lasix, and Carla will be drawing blood for serum electrolytes to determine her potassium level. Upon arrival at Mrs. Carroll's house, Carla discovers she does not have a tourniquet in her equipment bag. She is concerned about Mrs. Carroll because she is dyspneic, has 3+ edema in her lower legs, and complains of being very weak. What should she do?

List three items from Carla's bag or the client's home that could be used as a tourniquet:

_____

_____

_____

Rather than returning to the home health agency for a tourniquet and delaying client treatment, Carla could use a blood pressure cuff, rubber gloves, a piece of elastic, or a belt to obtain the blood sample. Being able to think creatively is an important skill for a nurse, not only as a time saver, but also as a means of cost containment and more expeditious client care.

Is creativity a trait we all possess? Are certain people born with more creativity than others? Clearly, there are those individuals who demonstrate more artistic ability than the rest of the general population, but this does not mean that we cannot all stretch our minds past what is commonplace and develop something new and different in a given situation.

We discussed the attributes of a critical thinker earlier in this chapter. Creative thinking builds on critical thinking: It requires the ability to think critically and the capacity to look at and analyze all angles of a situation to find a new or unique solution. It involves taking what is already known and using it in expanded ways—exactly what you, as an LPN/LVN moving to the RN level, are learning to do. In order to become a more creative thinker, you must be willing to break out of established patterns and look at things in a different way (Rubenfeld and Scheffer, 1995). Old habits must be evaluated and reshaped into new patterns. Creative thinking is important because it provides nurses with another means of solving problems when no obvious solution is available.

Whether you know it or not, you already use creative thinking each time you formulate a plan of nursing care for a client. When you use a scientific knowledge base to adapt care in each situation to the specific client, you are using creativity to individualize the care. But can nurses learn to become better creative thinkers? Box 6–2 describes one method that may be used to practice creative thinking. By practicing this as a skill, nurses may become more proficient at thinking creatively.

Box 6-2 Creative Thinking Practice

Steps for practicing creative thinking:*

1. Think of all current ways of viewing an idea, activity, etc.
2. Brainstorm all ways that could possibly replace current ways of viewing the idea, performing the activity, etc.
3. List pros and cons for all ideas and why they will or will not work
4. Imagine possible outcomes for each idea
5. Select one idea to use
6. Evaluate the outcome

* Practice using an activity with which you are familiar, say tying your shoes. See if you can find a new, creative approach to the activity.

The ability to think creatively helps nurses to be more productive members of a multidisciplinary health care team. This means that more ideas are generated to help the group achieve its goals. Client care can then become more specific and individualized when new approaches to solving problems are found. The registered nurse who is willing to think beyond established patterns in order to produce better solutions for client care is a definite asset in today's cost-conscious health care climate.

PROBLEM SOLVING

Problem solving is a thinking skill that may be used in all aspects of life, from personal situations to work-related matters. It is a component of critical thinking; that is, problem solving thinking processes are used during critical thinking. So it would seem apparent that a critical thinker must possess problem solving skills along with creative thinking abilities.

Problem solving may be defined as working out a correct solution to a problem or, more specifically to nursing, as "the process used to resolve or answer a proposed question or achieve an answer to a client need" (Klaasens, 1992). This skill typically has been incorporated into nursing education programs in the form of the nursing process (see chapter 7), but has not necessarily been taught as an independent thinking skill that may be applied to all aspects of client care.

For example, nurse managers are confronted with personnel and staffing concerns that require sound problem solving skills, and staff nurses are frequently involved in situations of an ethical nature with clients. The nursing process has been taught as a method to plan client care based on specific client problems, and therefore does not always apply to other problems confronting nurses on a daily basis. Since problem solving is important in all areas of nursing, it may be helpful initially to learn to use the skill independent of application to client care, or separate from the nursing process.

Let's first consider what is involved in the problem solving process. Various authors have described numerous steps to problem solving, but for our purposes the following process will be used:

- collection of data related to the problem
- identification and clarification of the problem
- exploration and evaluation of possible solutions
- selection of an appropriate solution
- implementation of the solution
- evaluation of the results

To learn to use these steps to problem solving, let's begin with application to everyday life. We are each presented with challenges to our routines that threaten to upset even the best laid plans; consider the following scenario.

You are a nursing student in an LPN to RN bridge program. It is 6:00 AM and you have just been awakened by a loud crash from the kitchen in your home. Upon investigation you discover that your cat has gotten into a cabinet and overturned a jar of insecticide and noxious fumes are filling the house. You have a class beginning at 7:00 AM, in which you are scheduled to take a midterm exam. Your spouse has already left for work, and you are alone at home.

Imagine yourself in this scenario. There is clearly a serious problem here. Using the problem solving process, list the steps you would take to arrive at a solution.

_____

_____

_____

_____

_____

_____

Can you see how problem solving is important in your personal life as well as in nursing? Now let's look at a client care situation in which the steps of the problem solving process may be used:

Dolly, a 63-year-old waitress, was in an automobile accident while she was driving intoxicated. She suffered a mangled leg, which had to be amputated. She has been very quiet and withdrawn since surgery, and refuses to get out of bed or wear her prosthetic leg to practice walking. The skin on her back is beginning to break down.

Use the problem solving process to identify this client's primary problem and list possible solutions, underlining the ones you would implement with this client:

_____

_____

_____

_____

_____

_____

Does the problem solving process seem easier with repeated practice? Hopefully, you are beginning to see that problem solving is a thinking skill that is very handy in nursing, and not only for client care planning. Think about its use in conflict resolution, such as in the following scenario:

> You are the nurse manager of a busy ICU and have just arrived at work to find the unit at full capacity and a note informing you that three nurses have called in sick. The chief of the medical staff calls to request that you attend his monthly medical chart audit meeting, since most of the patients to be reviewed are in ICU. As you attempt to explain your staff shortage, he becomes angry and threatens to have you fired unless you attend the meeting.

Identify the problem(s) in this scenario. Describe how the problem solving process may be used to find a solution to the conflict between the nurse and physician:

_____

_____

_____

_____

_____

_____

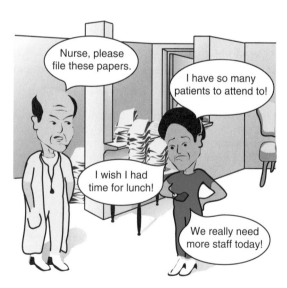

Figure 6-3
The problem solving process applies to all aspects of client care.

When more than one problem is identified, it may be necessary to prioritize and address the most important first. In the above scenario, client safety should take precedence over conflict between staff members. However, routine use of thinking skills prepares the nurse to sort through and address many issues in a short period of time.

All too often, nurses focus on the "doing" aspects of client care instead of using the analytical processes of problem solving (Hurst, Dean, and Trickey, 1991). When practiced as a thinking skill, problem solving will become more routine, and will be easier to apply in all areas of nursing (Figure 6–3). As a registered nurse, you will be expected to be able to quickly use effective problem solving skills when confronted with complex client care situations.

DECISION MAKING

Have you ever been in a situation in which you had to make a decision that could have very serious consequences for yourself and/or others? Decision making involves making a selection of actions to achieve a particular outcome (Pesut and Herman, 1999). Human beings often choose solutions that have worked in the past instead of considering the pros and cons of all possible choices. Registered nurses are frequently faced with making such decisions, and must be very adept at using an organized framework of thinking.

Various decision making models are described in the literature, such as the seven-stage format of Carroll and Johnson (1990). The stages are:

- recognition
- formulation
- alternative generation
- information search
- judgment or choice
- action
- feedback

You may notice that this framework seems similar to that of the problem solving process. There are fundamental differences, as the problem solving process involves taking steps to solve a particular problem and decision making is a thinking process for choosing the best action for a desired goal (Wilkinson, 1996).

According to Marquis and Huston (1992), decision making occurs after a known problem has already been identified, and emphasis should be placed on formulation of clear, specific goals. Their decision making framework includes the following:

- determination that a decision has to be made
- setting clear objectives (goals)

- searching for alternatives (by identifying all possible choices)
- evaluating alternatives (using logical, unbiased thinking)
- choosing a decision
- implementing the decision
- evaluating the results

Decision making differs from problem solving, which is an attempt to find a solution to eliminate the problem; however, decision making does not always solve the problem. In many instances a decision merely needs to be made to remedy a situation quickly; more time may then be devoted later to actual problem solving.

At this point you may be wondering how to keep frameworks for problem solving and decision making separate in your mind. You may also wonder if

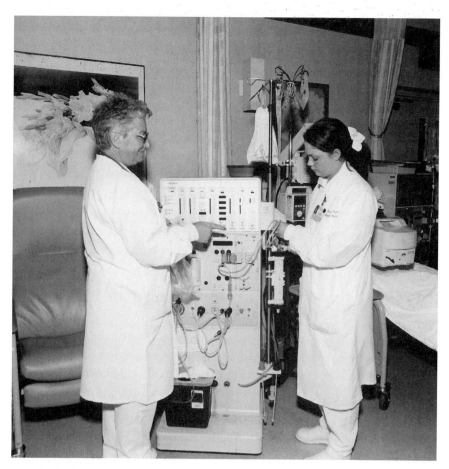

Figure 6-4
Registered nurses rely on knowledge and intuition for decision making.

you will remember to use all the correct steps when problems arise and decisions must be made. In truth, very few of us are consciously aware of using particular models when making decisions. By learning more about the thinking behind how we make decisions, we can improve clinical judgment. With practice, you will begin to subconsciously organize your thinking processes into a decision making framework when presented with a need to make a decision.

Let's consider the role personal instincts and judgment play in decision making. We are all products of our past experiences and environments, and are influenced by our own value systems, individual preferences, and individual ways of thinking when making a decision. In nursing, we tend to develop a "sixth sense" with regard to client care concerns, and apply our nursing intuition toward decision making.

The novice nurse has had a lifetime of general experiences that assist in decision making; however, the more experienced nurse has developed nursing judgment by virtue of trial and error in difficult situations. Therefore, it would seem reasonable that a decision making framework for nursing should include a logical process for analyzing alternatives, as well as components of judgment and intuition. The registered nurse calls upon previous experiences, knowledge, and nursing intuition when setting goals, analyzing alternatives, and making a decision (Figure 6–4). When a decision is made and acted upon, the resulting evaluation process provides further experiences which will enhance future nursing judgment and decision making skills.

Your ability to use decision making effectively as a thinking skill depends to a great extent upon your willingness to analyze personal decision making habits. Through the use of metacognition, you will gain insight into strengths and weaknesses in this process. Remember that past experiences as to what has worked before can be very beneficial; however, the use of a critical thinking approach to analysis of alternatives will render a more effective decision.

APPLICATION OF THINKING SKILLS TO PRACTICE

As we have seen, critical thinking, creative thinking, problem solving, and decision making are different thinking skills, yet they have much in common. Critical thinking is merely a method of logical, organized, analytical thinking applied to your thinking process. Creative thinking involves "breaking away" from established thinking patterns to find a new way of accomplishing a task. Problem solving calls for careful analysis and clarification of a problem before setting out to find the solution, whereas decision making is more concerned with finding a course of action to ensure a positive outcome rather than solving the problem.

At this point it should be clear that these skills are very useful to the registered nurse on a daily basis. No one skill must necessarily fit a particular client care situation. For example, critical thinking and problem solving may both be helpful in clarifying an ethical dilemma involving a client, and the ability to think creatively may enhance the decision making process. No two nurses will use thinking skills in the same manner, nor will they apply them to situations in the same way. Remember that we all have come from different backgrounds and bring different experiences to be drawn upon when planning client care. Think about these skills as you go about caring for your clients, analyze your own patterns of thinking, and evaluate for ways to improve your thinking.

The registered nurse who is able to quickly practice the four thinking skills described in this chapter is a valuable asset to clients in a variety of health care settings. As nurses become more autonomous members of the multidisciplinary health care team, the use of clear, organized thinking will be essential.

CRITICAL THINKING EXERCISES

1. Describe a situation in which you were required to solve a personal problem. List the steps you took to solve the problem. Did you use an organized framework of thinking? How might you change your process of thinking?

    _____

    _____

    _____

    _____

    _____

    _____

2. Describe three ways in which creative thinking will assist you in providing more effective client care:

    _____

    _____

    _____

    _____

    _____

3. Describe a situation in which you used intuition to help make a decision. Was it based on scientific knowledge or past experience? Was it helpful? Why or why not?

    _____

    _____

    _____

4. Analyze your own critical thinking skills, based on information presented
    in this chapter. Where are your strengths and weaknesses? How can you
    go about becoming a better critical thinker?

REFERENCES

Alfaro-LeFevre, R. (1999). *Critical thinking in nursing: A practical approach* (2nd ed.).
    Philadelphia: W.B. Saunders.

Allen, C. (1997). *Nursing process in collaborative practice: A problem solving approach* (2nd
    ed.). Stamford, CT: Appleton and Lange.

Carroll, J.S., and E.J. Johnson (1990). *Decision research: A field guide.* Newbury Park,
    CA: Sage.

Ennis, R.H. (1987). A taxonomy of critical thinking dispositions and abilities. In *Teaching
    thinking skills: Theory and practice*, J. Baron and R. Sternberg, eds. New York: Freeman.

Hurst, K., A. Dean, and S. Trickey (1991). The recognition and non-recognition of
    problem solving stages in nursing. *Journal of Advanced Nursing* 16:1444–1455.

Jacobs, P., B. Ott, B. Sullivan, Y. Ulrich, and L. Short (1997). An approach to defining
    and operationalizing critical thinking. *Journal of Nursing Education* 36(1):19–22.

Klaasens, E. (1992). Strategies to enhance problem solving. *Nurse Educator* 17(3):28–31.

Lipman, M. (1988). Critical thinking—What can it be? *Educational Leadership* 46:38–43.

Marquis, B., and C. Huston (1992). *Leadership roles and management functions in nursing:
    Theory and application.* Philadelphia: J.B. Lippincott.

Paul, R. (1992). *Critical thinking: What every person needs to survive in a rapidly changing
    world.* (2nd ed.). Santa Rosa, CA: Foundation for Critical Thinking.

Pesut, D., and J. Herman (1999). *Clinical reasoning: The art and science of critical and creative
    thinking.* Albany: Delmar.

Rubenfeld, M., and B. Scheffer (1995). *Critical thinking in nursing: An interactive approach.*
    Philadelphia: J.B. Lippincott.

Swartz, R., and D. Perkins (1990). *Teaching thinking: Issues and approaches.* Pacific Grove,
    CA: Midwest Publications.

Wilkinson, J. (1996). *Nursing process: A critical thinking approach.* (2nd ed.). Menlo Park,
    CA: Addison-Wesley Nursing.

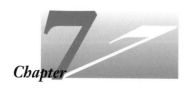

Chapter

Nursing Process:
A Framework
for Problem Solving

LEARNING OBJECTIVES

After completing this chapter, you will be able to:

1. Discuss three advantages to the use of an organizing framework for client care.
2. Compare the nursing process to the scientific method of problem solving.
3. Utilize the nursing process to assist the client and family in care planning.
4. Describe the relationship between critical thinking and the nursing process.

Collaborative Problem

North American Nursing Diagnosis Association (NANDA)

Nursing Diagnosis

Nursing Interventions Classification (NIC)

Nursing Outcomes Classification (NOC)

Nursing Process

Objective Data

Subjective Data

 Maria, Kevin, and Suzanna are taking time out from studying to walk in a local park.

Kevin: I'm really glad to have you two to talk to this year. My ex-wife is thinking about moving to another city and I'm afraid I won't be able to see my daughter as much as before. We have so much stress from school, and now this! It's nice to have friends who are willing to listen.

Maria: I know how you feel. I'd be devastated if I lost my children for even part of the time! Can you talk with your daughter's mother? Maybe you and she can work out something so the two of you can share custody. Remember the steps of the problem solving process . . . the ones we just discussed in our last nursing lecture? Maybe that would work now. How about drawing out a plan on paper that would suit everyone's needs?

Suzanna: Great idea, Maria! We really can apply thinking skills to everyday life. That lecture helped me see that. I'm looking forward to our next discussion, too—the one on the nursing process. As an LPN, I'm used to gathering client information and contributing to the client's care plan, but I still get confused about nursing diagnoses. The terminology seems so foreign to me sometimes!

Since the time of the earliest organized nursing orders, attempts have been made to identify the essence of nursing. More than a century ago, Florence Nightingale observed that "the very elements of nursing are all but unknown." Today, nurses are continuing efforts to define a body of knowledge and activities that make up nursing. In order to accomplish this complex task, a common language must be spoken among nurses. Perhaps the most frequently used method of communication is the nursing process.

During the 1950s, the nursing process was introduced as a mechanism to incorporate problem solving and decision making skills into a nursing care format. Based on the scientific method, the original nursing process framework involved a three-step process of assessment, planning, and evaluation. As the health care industry has become more outcomes-oriented, the nursing process has evolved into a five-step framework that includes assessment, diagnosis, planning, implementation, and evaluation.

In 1980, the American Nurses' Association (ANA) Social Policy Statement defined nursing as "the diagnosis and treatment of human responses to actual or potential health problems." Human responses include physiological, psychological, social, or spiritual reactions to an event or stressor (Wilkinson, 2000). In other words, nurses address a client's needs in a holistic manner. A later revision of the statement expanded nursing activities to encompass the full range of human experiences and responses to health and illness (American Nurses' Association, 1995).

During your practical/vocational nursing program, you were introduced to the nursing process. You practiced using the framework as a basis for organizing client care. As a registered nurse, you will be responsible for performing a comprehensive client assessment in order to formulate a plan of care, and will be much more involved in formulating nursing diagnoses and developing and evaluating client outcomes. The activities described in this chapter will guide you in the use of the nursing process, a systematic method of organizing client care.

WHY USE AN ORGANIZING FRAMEWORK?

Suppose you based nursing care simply on meeting immediate client needs and did not address problems in a systematic manner. In that case, there would be no continuity of care from one nurse to the next, and it would be difficult to establish and meet desired client outcomes. The **nursing process** is an organizing framework for client care activities that allows the nurse, client, and family to work together toward meeting established goals. The advantages of using the nursing process include:

- communication of the plan of care
- individualized client care
- client involvement
- nursing autonomy

By using the common language identified in the steps of the nursing process, nurses are able to clearly communicate the plan of care to co-workers. Everyone involved in a client's care—including the client and family—is addressing the same problems and is working toward the same outcomes. Documentation of client responses to interventions allows for evaluation and revision of care on a daily basis.

In today's managed care environment, clients are frequently placed on critical pathways (chapter 9) upon entry into a health care facility. Developed to standardize care for the common, most prevalent diagnoses, critical pathways do not allow for individualized client care. The steps of the nursing process provide a means for you, the nurse, to focus on individual client responses to health or illness. Based on the problem solving process, the nursing process incorporates an interpersonal, individualized approach to care. Two clients may have the same diagnosis, but require individualized nursing care plans that address needs unique to each. Holistic nursing care is more achievable with individualized care planning.

Use of the nursing process requires a collaborative effort among the nurse, the client, the family, and other health care team members. By encouraging client participation in care planning, the nurse fosters compliance and ensures customer satisfaction (Murray and Atkinson, 2000). Active involvement in care planning helps clients retain a sense of independence, rather than being passive recipients of care.

The nursing process provides you with the opportunity to exercise professional autonomy. Nursing is more than giving medications, assisting physicians, and changing dressings. The nursing process sets the stage for activities that involve thinking as well as doing (Figure 7–1). Use of the nursing process allows

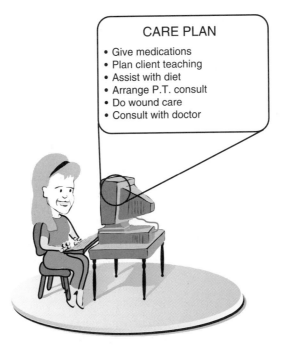

Figure 7–1
The nursing process involves both cognitive and psychomotor skills.

you to make independent decisions and maintain control of the profession. This results in greater job satisfaction and professional growth.

In summary, the nursing process is what nurses do. It helps clients, families, employers, and policy makers to understand what it is that nurses do. The process itself allows nurses and clients to use an organized framework to identify problems, plan outcomes and activities to restore health, and evaluate progress toward goals. It provides for consistent, client-centered, individualized care that empowers nurses to make independent decisions. The nursing process combines the science and the art of nursing; that is, it allows nurses to analyze and evaluate data to make decisions, as well as use intuition and judgment (Pesut and Herman, 1999). It can be used in any setting, with any group of people, and for any type of human response to health and illness. In summary, the nursing process:

- promotes continuity of care for clients
- provides a common framework of practice for nurses
- is planned and outcome-oriented
- fosters critical thinking
- involves input from the client and family
- is applicable to any client, regardless of setting, age, or diagnosis

THE STEPS OF THE NURSING PROCESS

Before the development of the term *nursing process*, the problem solving approach of John Dewey (1910) was used to guide clinical nursing. Many disciplines use a systematic problem solving framework; however, the nursing process utilizes knowledge drawn from nursing theories to make it unique. A side-by-side comparison of the nursing process and the problem solving process reveals similarities and differences, as shown in Table 7–1.

TABLE 7-1
Comparison of the Nursing Process to Problem Solving

NURSING PROCESS	PROBLEM SOLVING
Assessment	Identification of the problem
Diagnosis	Collection of data
Planning	Exploration of possible solutions
Implementation	Selection of a solution
	Implementation of the solution
Evaluation	Evaluation of results

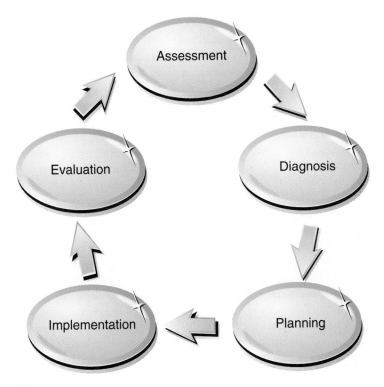

Figure 7–2
Cyclical nature of the nursing process.

The nursing process, however, has evolved into much more than a simple step-by-step guide to solving problems. Over the years, nurses have become more driven to formulate diagnoses from data, use critical thinking, and emphasize the unique caring nature of nursing (Murray and Atkinson, 2000). Today's five-step nursing process, shown in Figure 7–2, reflects the changing nature of the nurse–client relationship.

Assessment: Gathering Information

Assessment, the first step in the nursing process, consists of activities related to gathering information about the client, family, or community. Data collection provides a base upon which to proceed to other steps, and is ongoing. The nurse gathers physiological, psychological, sociocultural, developmental, spiritual, and environmental information about the client from various sources. Data obtained from the client are from a *primary source;* data gathered from the nurse, other health care staff, friends, and family are from *secondary sources.*

Nurses gather two types of data about clients: subjective and objective. Subjective data, sometimes called *symptoms*, come from the client directly, and describe feelings and perceptions. For example, a client's complaints of fatigue, dyspnea, nausea, and pain are examples of subjective information. Subjective data are personal and specific to the individual client, and cannot be experienced by the nurse.

Objective data, also known as *signs*, are observed by using the five senses, and are usually considered to be measurable. This information is obtained through observation and examination of the client. Examples of objective data are temperature, pulse, respiration, and blood pressure measurements taken by the nurse.

Nurses collect both subjective and objective data in order to get a complete picture of the client. If a client with pneumonia complains of "shortness of breath, weakness, and dizziness" (subjective data), the nurse could use laboratory test results (objective data) to begin identifying problems.

Various methods are used to collect client data, but those directly involving the client are the most helpful. The client interview (Table 7–2) consists of a one-to-one discussion between the nurse and client for the purpose of gathering baseline information about past and present health. A second client-centered method, the physical assessment, provides the nurse with objective data regarding the client's immediate health status. Nurses also gather information from friends and family of the client, medical records, and other health care team members.

Various nursing theorists have categorized client care needs into a format that may be helpful to the nurse when organizing assessment data. Two examples

TABLE 7-2
The Client Interview

Demographic information	Age, sex, marital status, educational level, employment status, and position
Chief complaint	Reason for seeking health care (in the client's own words)
History of the present illness	Events leading up to and contributing to the chief complaint
Past health history	Previous health problems, hospitalizations, surgeries, medications taken
Family health history	Health problems in family members, such as diabetes, heart disease, hypertension
Lifestyle habits	Alcohol consumption, nicotine use, caffeine intake, use of illegal drugs, dietary and exercise habits, sleep patterns
Psychosocial history	Support systems, coping pattern, spiritual practices, psychological history
Review of systems	Body systems data from client, any related difficulties
Home care needs	Cleanliness and safety factors, need for equipment, caregiver, transportation

are Marjorie Gordon's Functional Health Patterns (1999) and Virginia Henderson's 14 Nursing Problems (1966). As client information is gathered, it is placed under the appropriate category, where the nurse can begin to identify any areas of actual or potential problems. Table 7–3 is a comparison of the two formats.

Suppose, for example, you are the nurse who is admitting a diabetic client to your medical nursing unit. While taking a health history, you discover that the client has not been adhering to his diet. He complains of feeling thirsty, anorexic, and very tired.

Where would you place each of these items of information under Gordon's Functional Health Patterns? Under Henderson's 14 Nursing Problems?

_____

_____

_____

_____

_____

_____

TABLE 7–3
Client Care Needs

GORDON'S FUNCTIONAL HEALTH PATTERNS	HENDERSON'S 14 NURSING PROBLEMS
Health perception/health management	Breathe normally
Nutritional/metabolic	Eat and drink adequately
Elimination	Eliminate body waste
Activity/exercise	Move and maintain desirable posture
Cognitive/perceptual	Sleep and rest
Sleep/rest	Select clothing, dress and undress
Self-perception/self-concept	Maintain body temperature
Role/relationship	Cleanliness, grooming, skin integrity
Sexuality/reproductive	Avoid injury
Coping/stress tolerance	Communicate with others
Value/belief	Worship according to faith
	Take pride in chosen work
	Participate in recreation
	Health promotion activities

Once all pertinent data have been collected and grouped, the nurse should assess for accuracy. Information gathered from secondary sources (other than directly from the client) should always be verified, if possible.

Analysis: Determining the Problem

The second step of the nursing process begins with analysis of data collected during the assessment phase. Nurses cluster the data so that problems can be identified and nursing diagnoses formulated. This process of problem identification uses diagnostic reasoning (a form of clinical judgment) in which judgments, decisions, and conclusions are made about the meaning of the data collected. Following problem identification, nursing diagnoses are developed.

Even though nurses have been identifying and treating client problems since the beginning of the profession, the term *diagnosis* was primarily used by physicians until the early 1970s. At that time, a group of nursing leaders from the United States and Canada met in 1973 to develop a classification system of standard terminology and format for nursing diagnoses. The North American Nursing Diagnosis Association (NANDA) revises the original list of nursing diagnoses every two years. All nursing diagnoses are tested by nurses in actual practice, and are supported by defining characteristics, or signs and symptoms (Norwood, 1997). Box 7–1 contains a current listing of NANDA-approved nursing diagnoses.

Box 7-1   *NANDA Approved Nursing Diagnoses, 2001*

Activity intolerance	Breastfeeding, Effective
Activity intolerance, Risk for	Breastfeeding, Ineffective
Adjustment, Impaired	Breastfeeding, Interrupted
Airway clearance, Ineffective	Breathing pattern, Ineffective
Allergy response, Latex	Cardiac output, Decreased
Allergy response, Risk for latex	Caregiver role strain
Anxiety	Caregiver role strain, Risk for
Anxiety, Death	Comfort, Impaired
Aspiration, Risk for	Communication, Impaired verbal
Attachment, Risk for impaired parent/infant/child	Conflict, Decisional
	Conflict, Parental role
Autonomic dysreflexia	Confusion, Acute
Autonomic dysreflexia, Risk for	Confusion, Chronic
Body image, Disturbed	Constipation
Body temperature, Risk for imbalanced	Constipation, Perceived
	Constipation, Risk for
Bowel incontinence	Coping, Ineffective

Box 7-1 — NANDA Approved Nursing Diagnoses, 2001

Continued

Coping, Ineffective community
Coping, Readiness for enhanced community
Coping, Defensive
Coping, Compromised family
Coping, Disabled family
Coping, Readiness for enhanced family
Denial, Ineffective
Dentition, Impaired
Development, Risk for delayed
Diarrhea
Disuse syndrome, Risk for
Diversional activity, Deficient
Energy field, Disturbed
Environmental interpretation syndrome, Impaired
Failure to thrive, Adult
Falls, Risk for
Family processes: alcoholism, Dysfunctional
Family processes, Interrupted
Fatigue
Fear
Fluid volume, Deficient
Fluid volume, Excess
Fluid volume, Risk for deficient
Fluid volume, Risk for imbalanced
Gas exchange, Impaired
Grieving
Grieving, Anticipatory
Grieving, Dysfunctional
Growth and development, Delayed
Growth, Risk for disproportionate
Health maintenance, Ineffective
Health-seeking behaviors
Home maintenance, Impaired
Hopelessness
Hyperthermia
Hypothermia
Identity, Disturbed personal

Incontinence, Functional urinary
Incontinence, Reflex urinary
Incontinence, Stress urinary
Incontinence, Total urinary
Incontinence, Urge urinary
Incontinence, Risk for urge urinary
Infant behavior, Disorganized
Infant behavior, Readiness for enhanced organized
Infant behavior, Risk for disorganized
Infant feeding pattern, Ineffective
Infection, Risk for
Injury, Risk for
Injury, Risk for perioperative—positioning
Intracranial, adaptive capacity, Decreased
Knowledge, Deficient
Loneliness, Risk for
Memory, Impaired
Mobility, Impaired bed
Mobility, Impaired physical
Mobility, Impaired wheelchair
Nausea
Neglect, Unilateral
Noncompliance
Nutrition: less than body requirements, Imbalanced
Nutrition: more than body requirements, Imbalanced
Nutrition: more than body requirements, Risk for imbalanced
Oral mucous membrane, Impaired
Pain, Acute
Pain, Chronic
Parenting, Impaired
Parenting, Risk for impaired
Peripheral neurovascular dysfunction, Risk for

Box continued on following page

Box 7-1   *NANDA Approved Nursing Diagnoses, 2001*

Continued

Poisoning, Risk for
Post-trauma syndrome
Post-trauma syndrome, Risk for
Powerlessness
Powerlessness, Risk for
Protection, Ineffective
Rape-trauma syndrome
Rape-trauma syndrome, compound reaction
Rape-trauma syndrome, silent reaction
Relocation stress syndrome
Relocation stress syndrome, Risk for
Role performance, Ineffective
Self-care deficit, Bathing/hygiene
Self-care deficit
Self-care deficit, Feeding
Self-care deficit, Toileting
Self-esteem, Chronic low
Self-esteem, Situational low
Self-esteem, Risk for situational low
Self-mutilation
Self-mutilation, Risk for
Sensory perception, Disturbed
Sexual dysfunction
Sexuality patterns, Ineffective
Skin integrity, Impaired
Skin integrity, Risk for impaired
Sleep deprivation
Sleep pattern, Disturbed
Social interaction, Impaired

Social isolation
Sorrow, Chronic
Spiritual distress
Spiritual distress, Risk for
Spiritual well-being, Readiness for enhanced
Suffocation, Risk for
Suicide, Risk for
Surgical recovery, Delayed
Swallowing, Impaired
Therapeutic regimen management, Effective
Therapeutic regimen management, Ineffective
Therapeutic regimen management, Ineffective community
Therapeutic regimen management, Ineffective family
Thermoregulation, Ineffective
Thought processes, Disturbed
Tissue integrity, Impaired
Tissue perfusion, Ineffective
Transfer ability, Impaired
Trauma, Risk for
Urinary elimination, Impaired
Urinary retention
Ventilation, Impaired spontaneous
Ventilatory weaning response, Dysfunctional
Violence, Risk for other-directed
Violence, Risk for self-directed
Walking, Impaired
Wandering

The system developed by NANDA is congruent with ANA standards of practice and the 1995 ANA Social Policy Statement, all of which contribute to the move toward a common language in nursing. **Nursing diagnosis,** according to NANDA (2000), is "a clinical judgment about individual, family, or community responses to actual and potential health problems/life processes." Even though a client's medical diagnosis remains the same, nursing diagnoses may change as responses to illness or wellness change.

Nursing diagnoses are problems or responses that are primarily treated by nurses, and consist of four types: (1) actual, (2) risk (potential), (3) possible, and (4) wellness responses. Following is a brief description of each with examples:

1. *Actual* problems are existing responses to an event or stressor, such as illness. Examples are pain, fear, and knowledge deficit. Signs and symptoms must be present to support the problem.
2. *Risk (potential)* problems are of concern to the nurse because they may occur if actions are not taken to prevent them. For example, a client with weakness would be at risk for injury. Therefore, nursing interventions would be aimed at preventing falls.
3. A *possible* nursing diagnosis statement is used when a nurse does not have enough data to document an actual problem, but suspects that one exists. For example, a client who has just been told she has cancer might appear quiet and withdrawn. If a nurse suspects the client is experiencing fear of death, she would need to obtain more data in order to formulate an actual nursing diagnosis of death anxiety.
4. A *wellness* nursing diagnosis is used when the client exhibits a healthy response or strength. Effective breastfeeding is a wellness nursing diagnosis, describing a positive client response to a healthy state. These nursing diagnoses are used for clients who enjoy a relatively healthy level of wellness, but who would benefit from nursing interventions that will help them move to a higher level of wellness (Alfaro-LeFevre, 1998; Carpenito, 2000; Wilkinson, 2000).

A commonly used method of writing nursing diagnoses is the PES method, that is, the problem–etiology–signs and symptoms format (Figure 7–3). The first portion, or problem statement, is the NANDA label that describes the response, such as *pain*. The etiology consists of the causative factor(s) and begins with "related to," such as *related to lumbosacral muscle spasms*. The signs and symptoms are derived from the data base, such as *facial grimacing and voiced complaints*, and are preceded by "as evidenced by."

Actual problems have a three-part statement. Risk problems, however, have two parts because there are no supporting data indicating an actual problem. Possible nursing diagnoses are also two-part statements composed of the nursing diagnosis and related data that suggest a problem. Wellness diagnoses are expressed as single-part statements and describe an opportunity for enhanced health. Following are examples of diagnostic statements utilizing the PES format:

Actual Problem: Pain related to lumbosacral muscle spasms as evidenced by facial grimacing and voiced complaints
Risk Problem: Risk for infection related to lack of knowledge of sterile dressing change procedure

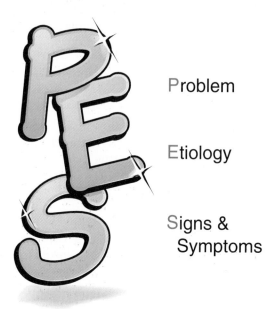

Figure 7-3
PES method of nursing diagnosis development.

> *Possible Nursing Diagnosis:* Possible altered parenting related to absence of
>   family support systems
> *Wellness Diagnosis:* Potential for enhanced health-seeking behaviors

If you are just beginning to learn to write nursing diagnoses, the task may
seem overwhelming. The terminology may seem like a foreign language, and
two- and three-part statements can become lengthy. With practice, the use of
nursing diagnoses will become easier and less confusing. There are, however,
several common errors you should avoid:

- Do not use a medical diagnosis as the causative factor:
  Incorrect: Fear related to appendectomy
  Correct: Fear related to uncertain outcome of surgical procedure
- Do not use a nursing diagnosis as the causative factor:
  Incorrect: Constipation related to impaired physical mobility
  Correct: Constipation related to limited activity secondary to frac-
  tured legs
  (note that a medical diagnosis is sometimes used, as here, to add clarity
  to the statement, in which case it is preceded by the phrase "secondary to")
- Do not use statements that are judgmental or legally inadvisable:
  Incorrect: Noncompliance related to poor attitude regarding self-care

Correct: Noncompliance related to lack of understanding of healthy life-style

- Do not write in terms of client needs or nursing interventions:
  Incorrect: Ineffective airway clearance related to need for frequent suctioning
  Correct: Ineffective airway clearance related to thick tracheobronchial secretions

From previous experience, you are familiar with medical diagnoses. Now you may be wondering if there is a relationship between nursing diagnoses and medical diagnoses. Actually, they address different aspects of client care. Medical diagnoses describe specific pathophysiological conditions, whereas nursing diagnoses are clinical judgements about client responses to illness. This does not mean that physicians and nurses do not have a common ground for addressing client needs. In fact, they often work together on a collaborative problem—a problem which occurs in relation to a physiologic condition, and which may be treated by various health care team members cooperatively. An example of a collaborative problem is a post-operative wound infection.

Nursing diagnoses provide nurses with a classifation system for client responses, and are the basis for the development of client goals, or expected outcomes. The next step of the nursing process sets the stage for the development of the nursing care plan.

Planning: Setting Goals and Choosing Nursing Actions

The third phase of the nursing process consists of two parts—(1) writing client goals and (2) planning interventions to help achieve those goals (Figure 7–4). The nurse, client, family, and other members of the health care team should work collaboratively to set client-specific goals in order to encourage compliance

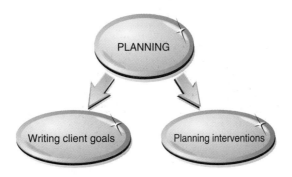

Figure 7–4
The planning phase consists of two parts.

with the plan of care (Leahy and Kizilay, 1998). It is during this phase of the nursing process that the nursing care plan is developed.

Historically, care plans have been handwritten documents that addressed client problems, goals, and interventions (Carpenito, 2000). Today, many health care agencies use computerized care plan formats that may be adapted to each client's needs. A care plan helps individualize care, improves continuity of care, and provides a means to evaluate goal achievement.

Before goals and interventions are developed into a plan of care, priority nursing diagnoses must be identified. The number of nursing diagnoses on the problem list depends on the type of client and health care setting. For a client who will receive care and be discharged within 24 hours, the list would probably be short. But for a client with complex problems requiring many interventions, some problems would have priority over others. One theoretical framework commonly used for prioritizing client problems is Maslow's Hierarchy of Needs (see chapter 4). In this system, basic physiological needs would take priority over physical safety, belonging, and self-esteem needs. Consider the following scenario:

> Dale is a 14-year-old who has sustained a gunshot wound to his face during a hunting accident. For the past three days, he has not been eating because of pain during chewing and swallowing. He complains of weakness, and frequently comments on his facial injury. He has lost weight and has difficulty breathing through his edematous nose. His nurse, Jessica, determines his problems to be:
>
> - Ineffective breathing patterns related to facial edema as evidenced by dyspnea
> - Body image disturbance related to facial wounds as evidenced by voiced concerns about scarring and future appearance
> - Altered nutrition: less than body requirements, related to verbalized dislike of food on bland diet as evidenced by weight loss

Using Maslow's theory as a basis for prioritizing needs, in which order should Dale's problems be ranked? Give your rationale:

_____

_____

_____

_____

_____

_____

It is unrealistic for nurses to expect to be able to address all client problems during the quick-turnover atmosphere in a modern-day health care agency. But by identifying priority diagnoses, the nurse can focus efforts on more immediate problems. Once a priority set of nursing diagnoses is established, outcome criteria may be developed.

Client goals, or outcomes, are statements about expected behavior or human responses after the implementation of nursing actions. They may fall into one of three categories: (1) cognitive (thinking), (2) affective (feeling), and (3) psychomotor (doing) behaviors (for further explanation, see chapter 8). Client outcomes should relate directly to each nursing diagnosis and should:

- contain action verbs
- be observable and measurable
- have a specified time limit

In addition, outcomes should be client-centered and realistic. An outcome does not state nursing actions; nor should it describe behavior that cannot be achieved. Outcomes should also be congruent with therapies planned by other health care team members (Murray and Atkinson, 2000). Following are the three nursing diagnoses used in the previous scenario, with examples of outcomes from each category:

1. *Nursing diagnosis:* Ineffective breathing patterns related to facial edema as evidenced by dyspnea
   Expected outcome: Client will maintain unlabored respirations at a rate of 12 to 20 during routine activities by time of discharge (psychomotor)
2. *Nursing diagnosis:* Body image disturbance related to facial wounds as evidenced by voiced concerns about scarring and future appearance
   Expected outcome: Client will verbalize rationale for treatment regimen prescribed to minimize scarring by second day of hospitalization (cognitive)
3. *Nursing diagnosis:* Altered nutrition: less than body requirements, related to verbalized dislike of food on bland diet as evidenced by weight loss
   Expected outcome: Client will demonstrate a willingness to use allowed dietary seasonings on foods by the second day of hospitalization (affective)

Outcomes may be written as either long- or short-term statements: *Long-term outcomes* reflect desired behavior at the end of care; *short-term outcomes* are achieved throughout the length of stay. As a student, you usually care for a client for a day or two at the most. Therefore, your client outcomes would more likely be short-term, and would be building blocks toward achievement of long-term outcomes.

A recent addition to the planning phase of the nursing process is the **Nursing Outcomes Classification (NOC),** first published in 1997. Based on client outcomes that are responsive to nursing care, NOC currently consists of 260 outcomes (Johnson, Maas, and Moorhead, 2000). This classification system offers several advantages:

- The outcomes are based on clinical nursing practice and research
- They may be shared by all disciplines

- The language is clear
- They address the entire scope of nursing practice

The NOC provides a standardized language for nursing to use in client care planning. Suppose you are caring for a female client who has been incontinent of urine each time she attempts to get up to the toilet. Following is an example of use of a NOC outcome:

Nursing Diagnosis: Urinary incontinence related to neuromuscular limitations as evidenced by inability to reach toilet before voiding
NOC Outcome: Demonstrates urinary continence, as evidenced by ability to successfully void in toilet

The suggested outcomes described by the NOC system are written in a language that is compatible with NANDA nursing diagnoses. They provide a way for nurses to communicate effectively with other health care professionals and explain the nature of nursing to the public (McCloskey and Bulechek, 2000).

After writing expected outcomes, the next step in planning is to develop specific nursing actions, or interventions, to aid the client in meeting the outcomes. Planned interventions include, but are not limited to, the following types of activities:

- ongoing assessment of the client
- client teaching about disease processes, treatments, medications, and so forth
- assistance with daily activities such as grooming, eating, and activity
- administration of medications
- performance of specific treatments to help resolve actual problems
- measures aimed at preventing complications or new problems
- collaboration with other health care professionals regarding plan of care

All nursing actions should be based on scientific principles, should be individualized to the client, and should specifically address etiology of the nursing diagnoses. Consider, for example, the following nursing diagnosis and expected outcome:

Nursing Diagnosis: Fluid volume deficit related to inadequate oral intake as evidenced by poor skin turgor, tachycardia, and complaints of thirst
Expected Outcome: Client will increase oral fluid intake to 1800 cc per day by discharge home

Nursing interventions aimed at achieving this outcome would therefore address measures to improve oral intake of fluids. Each nursing diagnosis and accompanying outcome should include a list of planned nursing interventions that specifically address the etiology of the problem.

The **Nursing Interventions Classification (NIC)** was first published in 1992, after clinically based research by a team of nurses from the University of

Iowa. It is a "comprehensive standardized language that describes treatments that nurses perform" (McCloskey and Bulechek, 2000, p. ix). Described as the nursing treatments of choice for each nursing diagnosis, NIC currently contains 486 interventions. Based on the previous example of the client with urinary incontinence, the following NIC intervention would be suggested: Assist the client with establishing a predictable pattern of bladder emptying in order to allow enough time to reach the toilet.

Both NIC and NOC may be used with NANDA nursing diagnoses and may follow standardized suggestions; each can still be individualized to each client. For a complete listing of current NIC and NOC interventions and outcomes, please refer to the publications listed in the references at the end of the chapter.

Implementation: Carrying Out the Plan

The fourth phase of the nursing process involves "applying the skills needed to implement the nursing interventions" (Carpenito, 2000, p. 69). Nurses communicate the plan of care to other health care team members through writing, verbal communication, and actual doing. During this phase, three types of nursing actions are used:

1. *Dependent:* Actions depend on orders from other professionals such as physicians; an example is a medication order
2. *Independent:* Actions ordered by nurses without direction from other professionals, such as turning a client every two hours to prevent skin breakdown
3. *Interdependent:* Actions mutually agreed upon by nurses and other health care professionals, such as a specific type of wound care

An essential step in the implementation phase is that of documentation of care. It is imperative that nurses record nursing actions and client responses in a timely manner in order to provide a basis for later evaluation activities (Figure 7–5). Methods of documentation vary with each agency, and nurses should become familiar with policies governing each.

Evaluation: Have Outcomes Been Met?

The final phase of the nursing process is evaluation, which involves determining the client's status based on whether expected outcomes have been achieved (Wilkinson, 2000). Evaluation is an ongoing process that can take place at any step in the nursing process. For example, interventions are evaluated by monitoring the client's response to nursing actions. Evaluation assists the nurse to decide which nursing actions are effective and which are not (Leahy and Kizilay, 1998).

Several sources may be used to determine whether outcomes have been met:

- direct observation of the client
- verbal communication with the client/family

- physical assessment of the client
- reports from other members of the health care staff
- review of lab reports, client records, and diagnostic test results

The nurse uses data gathered from these sources to determine whether outcomes have been (1) completely met, (2) partially met, or (3) not met at all. If expected outcomes have not been completely met, each step of the nursing process should be analyzed to see where modifications need to be made.

Failure to achieve expected outcomes completely may be due to one of several reasons. If the nurse has not collaborated with the client and family, goals may be unrealistic for the client to achieve. Perhaps the client was involved in care planning, but did not view the achievement of outcomes to be as important as other aspects of care.

Many times planned nursing interventions are not effectively communicated to other staff members, resulting in lapses in continuity of care. As client needs change from day to day, care plans are not always adjusted to reflect new problems.

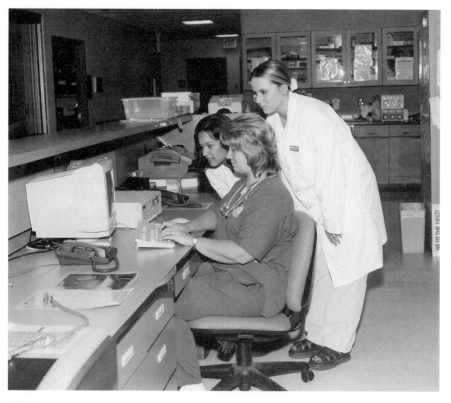

Figure 7–5
Documentation is an important part of the nursing process.

Ongoing evaluation of nursing care assists the nurse to revise care plans as necessary, rather than at the time of discharge. Feedback gathered from evaluation activities gives the nurse and client an opportunity to analyze decisions, actions, and behavior changes constructively, then implement further revised interventions if indicated.

CRITICAL THINKING AND THE NURSING PROCESS

Now that you've been introduced to the steps of the nursing process, you should note that actual care of clients does not always progress in a structured, orderly fashion. In reality, client care situations often present difficulties for even the most experienced nurse. Simply knowing how to use the nursing process does not guarantee effective management of complex client problems.

To ensure quality client care, it is imperative that you be able to use high level thinking and reasoning skills. Chapter 6 contains a description of thinking skills that are frequently utilized by nurses. Of the skills discussed, problem solving is perhaps the most closely related to each step of the nursing process.

During the assessment phase, nurses must be able to gather reliable data in order to identify appropriate problems. A critical thinker is one who can distinguish between relevant and irrelevant information (Wilkinson, 2000). Care is taken to ensure a thorough, complete history by the nurse who uses critical thinking. In addition, the nurse utilizes a wide variety of sources for data collection, and resists making assumptions about client problems until credibility of data is assured.

During the diagnosis phase of the nursing process, nurses need to be able to form sound conclusions based on available information. When thinking critically, relationships between bits of information are analyzed and tentative inferences are made in the form of nursing diagnoses. Gaps in data are noted and inconsistencies are recognized as the nurse attempts to state each problem as clearly and completely as possible.

When planning care, the critical thinker uses scientific/nursing theories (see chapter 4) upon which to base expected outcomes and suggested interventions. Established principles are used to support chosen nursing actions, rather than relying on unproven opinions.

As the plan of care is implemented, the critical thinker continuously strives to include all necessary actions to help the client achieve planned outcomes. Creativity may be used to solve unexpected difficulties during this phase of the nursing process. Decisions are made after careful deliberation.

Finally, during the evaluation phase of the nursing process the nurse very carefully analyzes client responses to determine effectiveness of care. If goals have not been met, the critical thinker asks what went wrong and begins thinking of ways to revise the plan of care in an open-minded manner.

Critical thinking involves using sound judgment and logic. Nurses who practice critical thinking during client care are less likely to accept false assumptions and wrong data. The nursing process provides an excellent format for the nurse to exercise critical thinking skills.

In summary, the nursing process is a systematic, cyclic process whereby each step leads to the next, yet also relates to all others. Use of the nursing process ensures "consistent, comprehensive, and coordinated" care (Norwood, 1997). As you move from practical/vocational to registered nursing, you will find the nursing process to be an excellent means of communicating what you do as a nurse to clients, the community, and other health care professionals.

CRITICAL THINKING EXERCISES

1. Compare and contrast the nursing process and the scientific method of problem solving. How is the nursing process unique?

_____

_____

_____

_____

_____

_____

2. Use a case study or actual client for whom you have provided nursing care to do an assessment interview. Group data according to Gordon's Functional Health Patterns. How does this exercise differ from care planning you have done as a practical/vocational nurse?

_____

_____

_____

_____

_____

_____

3. Do you believe the nursing process is an effective means to communicate to others about what nurses do? Why?

_____

_____

_____

_____

_____

_____

4. Using the client example from question 2, formulate three priority nursing diagnoses. Develop at least one expected outcome for each.

_____

_____

_____

_____

_____

_____

REFERENCES

Alfaro-LeFevre, R. (1998). *Applying nursing process: A step-by-step guide* (4th ed.). Philadelphia: Lippincott.

American Nurses' Association. (1995). *Nursing's social policy statement.* Washington, D.C.

Carpenito, L. (2000). *Nursing diagnosis: Application to clinical practice* (8th ed.). Philadelphia: Lippincott.

Dewey, J. (1910). *How we think.* New York: D.C. Heath.

Gordon, M. (1999). *Manual of nursing diagnosis.* St. Louis: C.V. Mosby.

Henderson, V. (1966). *The nature of nursing: A definition and its implications for practice, research, and education.* New York: Macmillan.

Johnson, M., M. Maas, and S. Moorhead (2000). *Nursing Outcomes Classification (NOC)* (2nd ed.). St. Louis: C.V. Mosby.

Leahy, J., and P. Kizilay (1998). *Foundations of nursing practice: A nursing process approach.* Philadelphia: W.B. Saunders.

McCloskey, J., and G. Bulechek (2000). *Nursing Interventions Classification (NIC)* (3rd ed.). St. Louis: C.V. Mosby.

Murray, M., and L. Atkinson (2000). *Understanding the nursing process in a changing care environment* (6th ed.). New York: McGraw-Hill.

North American Nursing Diagnosis Association (2001). *NANDA nursing diagnoses: Definitions and classification—2001–2002.* St. Louis.

Norwood, B. (1997). Essentials of the nursing process. In *Professional nursing: Concepts and challenges* (2nd ed.), K. Chitty, ed. Philadelphia: W.B. Saunders.

Pesut, D., and J. Herman (1999). *Clinical reasoning: The art and science of critical and creative thinking.* Albany: Delmar.

Wilkinson, J. (2000). *Nursing process: A critical thinking approach.* (3rd ed.). Menlo Park, CA: Addison-Wesley Nursing/Benjamin Cummings.

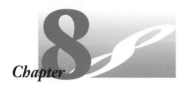

Chapter

The Educator Role of the Registered Nurse

LEARNING OBJECTIVES

After completing this chapter, you will be able to:

1. Discuss the importance of the teaching role of the registered nurse to client care.
2. Discuss principles of adult learning and their application to client education.
3. Discuss the importance of developmental considerations in client education.
4. Identify effective nursing strategies for dealing with barriers to client education.
5. Utilize the nursing process to formulate a client teaching plan.

Andragogy   Client Teaching Plan   Learning Barriers

Client Teaching   Knowledge Domains   Pedagogy

Maria, Kevin, and Suzanna are meeting at Kevin's apartment to work together on client care plans.

Suzanna: Are you as tired as I am? The nursing process seems pretty involved to me. I'm not really sure I see the need for all this written work. Why can't we just go to the hospital and take care of our clients without writing down what we plan to do? Our instructors want us to be able to interpret assessment data and plan for discharge teaching. I'm starting to feel comfortable with doing client assessments, but I've never done client teaching. Shouldn't we take classes on teaching techniques first?

Kevin: I've used the nursing process at work to plan care for my clients, but I have to admit I *am* learning to use it in more depth as an RN student. I also feel a little nervous about adding client teaching to my care plan, because I've never really been taught how to teach clients. When clients are discharged home while I'm at work, I give them their discharge instructions . . . the ones the doctor writes. But I don't usually think about teaching at other times.

Maria: I'm an LPN in a long-term care facility, so I don't usually get the chance to do much client teaching. And I don't do care plans in the format we're learning about in this nursing program. At this point the nursing process and client teaching seem pretty overwhelming to me. Even if I *do* learn this information, I'm not sure I'll ever use it at work.

Because they have such close association with clients, nurses are in an excellent position to provide health care information. Shorter hospital stays and changes in health care spending have made the need for client education critical. Recipients of health care can no longer check into a hospital for a routine illness and expect to stay until they are completely well. Clients and their families are being encouraged to take an active part in care from admission to discharge, including continuing home care. Consumers of health care have become increasingly aware that they actually have choices in life that may affect their general health, and are turning to health care professionals for answers to their questions.

These changes have created a role shift for registered nurses. Where nurses once served merely as advocates who clarified information for clients, they are currently playing an active part in a holistic approach to client education. As a registered nurse, you will be responsible for assessing client learning needs, formulating an individualized teaching plan, overseeing implementation, and evaluating the outcomes of teaching, regardless of the setting.

The practical/vocational nurse's part in client teaching involves implementation of the teaching plan at a basic health needs level (Hill and Howlett, 2001). Registered nurses, on the other hand, have the responsibility for providing education to clients, families, and communities, based on a comprehensive assessment of health care needs.

The purpose of this chapter is to explain the role of the registered nurse as a client teacher, with an emphasis on differences in the responsibilities of the registered nurse and the practical/vocational nurse. Acquiring a more extensive knowledge base about client care should help you to feel more prepared for client teaching; however, a discussion of teaching–learning principles is also in order if you are to develop client teaching plans effectively.

THE NURSE AS A TEACHER

When you first considered nursing as a career, did you know teaching would be a very large part of your duties? Most students entering nursing school do not realize how much time will be spent assessing learning needs and actually teaching clients, families, and others. Why, then, don't nurses take education courses while in nursing school? Practical/vocational nursing programs typically do not emphasize **client teaching** as a role of the LPN/LVN. Most registered nursing curricula incorporate client teaching principles into all areas of content. Nursing students are asked to implement individualized teaching strategies as they care for clients.

Various regulatory agencies have recognized the importance of client teaching. The American Nurses' Association (ANA), the Joint Commission on Accreditation of Healthcare Organizations (JCAHO), Medicare, Medicaid, and local state boards of nursing have mandated that nurses implement client teaching into their daily care plans. In addition, the Patients' Bill of Rights assures health care recipients of a complete explanation of their diagnosis and related treatment. It is essential, therefore, that you as a registered nurse be prepared to present health information to clients in a variety of settings, regardless of age, education, and cultural and socioeconomic needs (Leahy and Kizilay, 1998).

You may be wondering if you have what it takes to be an effective teacher. Take a few minutes to answer the following questions:

What personality characteristics do you think are essential in a good teacher?

_____

_____

_____

_____

_____

_____

Which of these characteristics do you possess? Which should you develop in order to be a more effective client teacher?

_____

_____

_____

_____

_____

_____

Box 8–1 lists several interpersonal skills important to the nurse who is a client teacher. In addition, it is imperative that the nurse be adept at evaluating the effectiveness of the teaching, make changes as needed in the teaching plan, and document outcomes appropriately.

Box 8-1   *Characteristics of the Nurse Teacher*

- Caring
- Supportive
- Competent
- Empathetic
- Attentive
- Professional
- Respectful
- Nonjudgmental

Whether you are explaining a procedure to help reduce a client's fears or conducting a formal educational program for a group of newly diagnosed diabetics, teaching is an inherent function of nursing. If the major goals of nursing are to prevent illness, promote or restore health, and facilitate coping with chronic and terminal illness, client teaching is a useful tool for accomplishing these tasks.

PRINCIPLES OF ADULT LEARNING

We have discussed the importance of client teaching from the nurse's standpoint, as well as characteristics of an effective teacher. But what about the client's willingness to learn? Are there factors that may have an impact on whether client learning actually takes place? Do all clients want to learn information related to their diagnosis and self-care? Do they all have the ability to learn?

Describe a situation in which you provided education to a client/family (either as an LPN/LVN or as a nursing student).

_____

_____

_____

_____

_____

_____

Was the client/family ready and willing to learn? Did you feel adequately prepared to answer all their questions?

_____

_____

_____

_____

_____

_____

If you have not had formal instruction in teaching theory and strategies, client teaching can be a little frightening. Perhaps a discussion of adult learning theory will provide useful information as to how adults learn.

One of the simplest ways to envision how adults learn is by grouping learning processes into three areas: (1) knowledge, (2) attitudes, and (3) skills. These categories are described in different terms by Bloom (1956), who classifies the three knowledge domains as cognitive (knowledge), affective (attitudes), and psychomotor (skills).

Within each learning domain we can develop specific learning objectives (expected outcomes) for our clients, as shown in Table 8–1. These learning objectives are the expected outcomes upon which the client's care plan is based.

As a practical/vocational nurse, you may already be involved in client teaching; however, the formulation of the teaching plan is typically the responsibility of a registered nurse. When developing a client teaching plan, you as the registered nurse must decide the domain within which the teaching should be focused. If, for example, a client needs to be taught signs and symptoms of hypoglycemia, your focus should be on cognitive, or knowledge level material. On the other hand, teaching an obese client the importance of adhering to a diabetic diet would fall into the affective category, because a change in attitude would be desirable. In this instance, your expected outcome would be for the client to express an interest in learning healthful eating habits.

Now let's pause briefly to consider the role of the practical/vocational nurse in client education. Generally, practical/vocational nurses are educated to identify client strengths and weaknesses regarding health care information, while registered nurses are taught to be responsible for formulating expected outcomes of learning. Practical/vocational nurses contribute important assessment data to the development of client teaching plans, and they assist with implementation of planned interventions. The registered nurse, however, has the primary respon-

TABLE 8-1
Examples of Client Behaviors in Bloom's Domains of Knowledge

COGNITIVE	AFFECTIVE	PSYCHOMOTOR
States side effects of medications	Expresses desire to learn about medications	Demonstrates self-administration of medications
Discusses rationale for taking own BP	Cooperative during demonstration of how to take own BP	Demonstrates how to take own BP
Discusses importance of breastfeeding infant	Appears happy to be breastfeeding infant	Successfully breastfeeds infant
Describes calorie restrictions of diabetic diet	Listens attentively to discussion about food exchanges on diabetic diet	Plans own daily menus from diabetic diet guidelines

sibility of identifying client learning needs, formulating nursing diagnoses, setting goals for client outcomes, overseeing the implementation of planned interventions, and evaluating the results.

Next let's consider characteristics of the adult learner. Up to this point, you may not have realized that adults learn differently than children. **Pedagogy** is the science and practice of teaching others. **Andragogy** is a form of pedagogy: It is the art of teaching as applied specifically to adults. Andragogy has been extensively studied by Malcolm Knowles (1984), who distinguishes adult learners from children as learners in the following ways:

1. Adults are self-directed learners; they are not as dependent on the teacher to decide what they need to learn.
2. Adults utilize past experiences to build a knowledge base, which can be used as a resource for future learning.
3. Adults link a readiness to learn to specific life-changing events, such as a job promotion or the birth of a baby.
4. Adults need to be able to apply material to be learned to real life events.
5. Adults like to take an active part in their own educational process.

In addition, several other characteristics of adult learners set them apart from children as learners. For example, adults do not have mandatory education past high school graduation, so their participation in learning is strictly voluntary. Adults generally expect to obtain information that will be useful to them, and may demand that teachers provide them with it. In many instances, adult learners may have more experience in certain situations than the teacher, and hence may challenge information provided in class (Redman, 1997). As a registered nurse, you must remember to take these aspects of adult learning into consideration when planning teaching. Table 8–2 includes a list of other teaching–learning principles and suggested nursing interventions that apply to adults. When planning client education, you should remember these characteristics specific to adult learners.

What about client teaching with children, adolescents, and the elderly? Adult learning principles do not specifically address these age groups. We need to remember that we may be asked to answer health care questions by clients and families who have members of different ages.

Infants and young children are not usually as involved in client education as older children and adolescents, but still need explanations about what is going to happen to them. You should work with the parents to plan outcomes, and provide education to young children at a simple, understandable level. In these age groups, children react strongly to procedures that cause discomfort, and need the support of a loved one. By including the support person in the child's education, much of the anxiety surrounding procedures may be diminished.

School-age children are curious about their diagnosis, tests, and medications. They are usually ready for direct formal teaching by the nurse. For example, a ten-year-old boy could be taught a short list of foods contained in a diabetic

TABLE 8-2
Adult Teaching–Learning Principles

PRINCIPLES	NURSING INTERVENTIONS
1. Learning should be personalized	1. Meet with client and family to determine individual learning needs
2. Climate should be conducive to teaching and learning	2. Make sure climate is comfortable and quiet; choose a private location
3. Organize information from simple to complex	3. Begin teaching plan with basic concepts to lay groundwork, then move to more difficult concepts as client understands
4. Active participation is essential if learning is to take place	4. Structure session so client and family have time for questions and to participate in their own learning
5. Learning is retained longer when it is put into immediate use	5. Allow client to use information from learning session immediately in own self-care
6. Learning is facilitated when the learner receives immediate feedback	6. Have client demonstrate new knowledge/skills and give immediate feedback
7. Personal values affect learning	7. Evaluate client's value system prior to teaching and structure lesson to be congruent with those values
8. Learning and change are stressful	8. Allow client time to voice concerns about changes which require education; remain supportive and available to assist as needed

diet. Children in this age group are beginning to understand cause and effect, so they can often grasp the consequences of their actions (Redman, 1997). Drug awareness programs, for example, are begun with school-age children.

Adolescents are mature enough to pay attention to details and to analyze problems (Leahy and Kizilay, 1998), and thus can participate in setting expected outcomes. They enjoy being given the freedom to make choices regarding when teaching sessions will take place. Adolescent clients are also at an age where they want to be like their peers; they do not want be seen as different, so you may find teaching somewhat challenging. A client teaching plan for an adolescent should be designed to allow for these special developmental considerations.

Elderly clients may have hearing, visual, and memory alterations that affect client teaching. It is important to thoroughly assess for any sensory or cognitive impairments prior to planning for teaching. Older adults may need teaching sessions at a time when they are best able to concentrate, and are not fatigued or uncomfortable (Leahy and Kizilay, 1998). Family members, especially those who will be primary caregivers, need to be included in teaching sessions, and ample time for questions should be provided.

FACTORS THAT MAY AFFECT THE LEARNING PROCESS

Several factors influence learning, some of which may actually be learning barriers (Box 8–2). Before any client teaching is implemented, nurses should make an assessment to determine whether the client (1) can learn, (2) is ready to learn, and (3) has a positive attitude toward learning (Leahy and Kizilay, 1998).

An educated client who has lived longer would clearly bring more life experiences and problem solving ability into a learning situation. A higher level of maturity and a strong support system have been shown to positively affect a client's readiness to learn. Previous experience with illness and health care professionals may also better prepare a client for learning.

Certain factors, however, can inhibit a client's ability to learn effectively, regardless of how well the information is presented. For example, stress over financial concerns, pain, and fear of a poor prognosis can distract a client from absorbing information that is not considered as important at that time (Figure 8–1). Cultural differences may interfere with a client's capacity to readily accept a particular method of self-care, and language barriers may cause information to be misunderstood.

A client may be eager to listen and learn about new information, or may choose not to participate in the discussion. Whichever is the case, you must be flexible enough to adapt the plan of care to continue to meet client needs. Sometimes this means looking for those "teachable moments," such as when a client asks why he is receiving a new medication, or when a new mother is unable to get her infant to breastfeed on the first attempt.

Box 8-2   *Factors Influencing Learning*

- Limited time for teaching/learning
- Educational level of learner
- Absence of support system
- Previous experience with illness
- Fear of prognosis
- Financial concerns
- Pain/physical discomfort
- Language barriers
- Cultural differences
- Altered mental processes

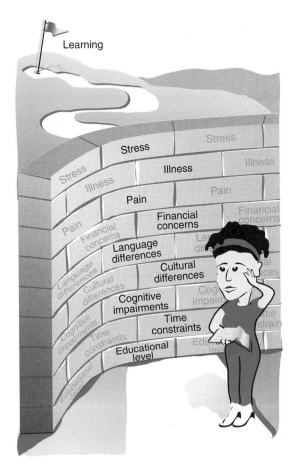

Figure 8–1
Learning barriers.

In order to overcome barriers to client learning, you must use good assessment skills to identify potential problems before the teaching plan is implemented (Smith, 1987). Consider the following scenario for example:

Jennifer, a 22-year-old, has been diagnosed with a kidney stone and is to undergo a lithotripsy procedure at 8:00 the following morning. Larry, the evening nurse on the medical-surgical nursing unit, is assigned to do teaching with Jennifer about the procedure. Upon entering her room, Larry finds Jennifer crying because she has had to leave her 6-month-old baby with her mother while she is hospitalized.

Is this a good time for the nurse to teach the client about her planned procedure? Please answer the following questions:

What barrier to learning is easily identifiable? What could the nurse do to ensure that the client is ready for learning?

_____

_____

_____

_____

_____

_____

We have already noted that stress may have a negative effect on learning. Obviously, in order to capture the attention of the client in the scenario, the nurse must first alleviate her anxiety about her child. When assessing a client's readiness to learn, you must always be mindful of factors that could impede learning. A **client teaching plan** must be flexible enough to allow for changes based on such factors.

THE PROCESS OF CLIENT TEACHING

The actual process of teaching a client may consist of a formal, planned session, or it may be as simple as a spur-of-the-moment answer to a question. If the thought of writing a sophisticated lesson plan for a client is rather overwhelming, be assured that the majority of client teaching takes place informally, and may not require a great deal of preparation.

Whether or not you choose to develop a formal written guide when teaching clients, a systematic approach to the activity is important. The process of client teaching can be outlined in the following steps:

1. Determine the client's need for education
2. Evaluate the client's readiness to learn
3. Prepare for teaching the client
4. Perform teaching activities with the client
5. Evaluate the client for learning

Let's look at each of these steps in turn.

Before any client teaching is performed, a thorough assessment must be carried out in order to identify specific learning needs. The nursing diagnosis most often used for clients who require teaching is *knowledge deficit* (see chapter

7). This deficit may be in one or more of the many areas in which clients need education, such as medications, diet, activity, disease process, diagnostic procedures, and self-care. For example, a newly diagnosed renal failure client and family may have a knowledge deficit regarding fluid and dietary restrictions. Prior to planning for client teaching, you must first determine what the client and family already know, and use that knowledge as a starting point.

Next the client's readiness for learning must be established. If barriers to learning exist, they must be taken into consideration and handled accordingly. The client and family must be evaluated for motivation and desire to learn, as these factors strongly affect retention of material being taught, as well as compliance with treatment. Learning goals must be congruent with the client's value system if cooperation and participation are to occur (Harrington, Smith, and Spratt, 1996).

Preparing for the teaching session should involve input from the nurse, client, and family/significant others. Individualized, specific goals should be developed as to the expected outcomes to be achieved after the teaching has occurred. These goals, or expected outcomes (see chapter 7), should contain action words, be measurable, and have a stated time frame within which to be met. Let's use the example of the newly diagnosed renal failure client and family to write expected outcomes for a nursing diagnosis of *knowledge deficit*:

Nursing Diagnosis: Knowledge deficit related to lack of understanding of fluid/dietary restrictions, as evidenced by a twenty-pound weight gain in three days.

Expected Outcome 1: Given a list of foods and beverages, the client will correctly identify those which are inappropriate for a renal diet before discharge home from the hospital (cognitive domain).

Expected Outcome 2: The client will maintain a weight gain of less than ten pounds between each triweekly clinic visit (psychomotor domain).

Note that the knowledge domains for the two expected outcomes have been identified to assist you to better under this concept. Before progressing to the next step of client teaching, you must be sure the established outcomes seem achievable to the client and others who will be assisting with care.

Preparation and planning for client teaching also involves gathering any information needed for teaching and finding a comfortable setting that is conducive to learning. Aids to learning may be helpful, as clients have different learning styles (Figure 8–2). Most health care agencies provide clients with written instructions for self-care upon discharge, which make your job much easier. Education guides, pamphlets, and handouts can supplement verbal instructions given by the nurse (Palmerini and Jasovsky, 1998). Anatomically correct models, videos, and computer programs are other teaching aids that are available for client education. Many clients learn better by actually being able to visualize a concept; they may, for instance, find it helpful to see a blocked coronary artery on a model.

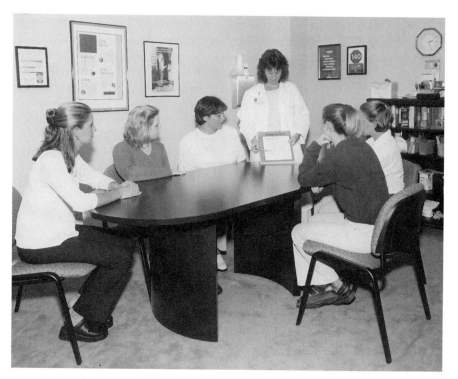

Figure 8–2
Nurses use learning aids to enhance client teaching.

If a psychomotor skill is to be taught, you should reserve sufficient time in your work schedule for demonstration and client practice. A client may feel overwhelmed when first learning a new skill, especially one involving new technology and terminology. By teaching the skill, allowing time for practice, then returning later for repeated practice, you can assist the client to assimilate the information in a nonthreatening manner.

The evaluation process of client education actually begins as you are presenting the new information. During the education session, be alert to cues from the client that would indicate an understanding of the material being taught. Clients should be addressed in a respectful, nonjudgmental manner, and information presented in language that is understandable. Frequent pauses for questions enable the learner to clarify material and understand it better. At the end of the session, a brief synopsis of pertinent principles will assist clients to retain information. It may be helpful to the client for you to return at a later time to answer any other questions that may have arisen, especially if family and friends arrive later.

The previously established expected outcomes should be evaluated at this point. If they have not been met, allow time to work with the client and family to make revisions that will promote success. And, finally, the process is not complete without proper documentation on the client care record as to the teaching performed and resulting outcomes.

As you may have already noticed, the steps described here in the process of client teaching closely resemble those of the nursing process (chapter 7). The following section will provide you with a sample client case study and teaching plan following the format of the nursing process.

APPLICATION OF CLIENT TEACHING TO THE NURSING PROCESS

After being introduced to adult learning principles, knowledge domains, characteristics of the effective nurse teacher, and barriers to learning, you may be wondering how you will be able to incorporate so much information into client teaching. Perhaps a look at client teaching using the nursing process will help you to visualize this activity with clients. The following case study incorporates concepts discussed in this chapter, and suggests one format for designing a client teaching plan:

CASE STUDY

Donna Adams is a 36-year-old who has a four-year history of diabetes mellitus. Her blood sugar has been well controlled on oral medication until recently; now she has been diagnosed with rheumatoid arthritis, which has caused hyperglycemic episodes. Donna has been admitted to the hospital for treatment of dehydration and stabilization of her blood sugar. In order to better regulate Donna's blood sugar, her doctor has placed her on regular insulin 8 units SQ each AM and NPH insulin 12 units SQ each PM. She lives in a low-income housing complex, is unemployed, and is raising her three children alone. Her parents live in a nursing home in another state, and are her only relatives besides her children.

Becky Randall is a day-shift nurse who has been assigned to care for Donna on the first day of her hospitalization. When she enters Donna's hospital room for her initial morning assessment, Donna says, "I'm so scared I won't be able to give my own shots. My kids rely on me to do so much for them, and now I'm sick."

Teaching Plan

I. *Assessment:* Becky collected the following data during an initial assessment of Donna:
   A. The need to better understand her illness and insulin requirements

    B. The need to learn self-administration of insulin

    C. Anxiety about giving injections to herself

    D. Concern about being too ill to care for her children

    E. Potential difficulty obtaining medical supplies because of financial status

    F. Lack of adult support system

II. *Diagnosis:* The following nursing diagnoses are formulated by Becky, based on the data collected in the assessment phase:

    A. Knowledge deficit (management of self-care) related to change in therapeutic regimen.

    B. Anxiety related to concern about ability to self-administer insulin and adequately care for children.

    C. Home maintenance management, risk for impairment, related to lack of financial resources for medical supplies and lack of support persons.

III. *Planning:* During this phase, Becky acts as a supportive, caring listener to assist Donna in planning expected outcomes to address the identified nursing diagnoses. From information obtained during the assessment phase, Becky anticipates that Donna's illness, stress level, and lack of family support could be barriers to learning. Therefore, as the acute illness is being stabilized, she spends time getting to know Donna and establishing a trusting relationship before formulating a teaching plan. The following expected outcomes are developed by Donna and Becky:

    A. By discharge from the hospital, Donna will correctly demonstrate self-administration of insulin.

    B. By the third day of hospitalization, Donna will verbalize improved feelings of ability to care for self and children.

    C. By discharge from the hospital, Donna will express satisfaction with plans for financial assistance for home care.

Becky and Donna agree to begin the teaching session on the third hospital day when the morning insulin dose is due. Becky organizes her other responsibilities around this time in order to spend about 20 minutes with Donna. Becky prepares for the session by refreshing her memory on the content to be presented and gathering supplies and handouts on diabetes and insulin administration.

IV. *Implementation:* Prior to beginning client teaching, Becky contacts a social worker to talk with Donna regarding resources available to help fund home care supplies, as well as possible help with her children. Becky and Donna decide to wait until Donna has worked out these concerns with the social worker before discussing insulin self-administration.

The following is an outline of the content that is presented to Donna by Becky during the education session:

    1. An initial overview of what the lesson will contain

    2. A brief explanation of changes in diabetes secondary to other diseases

      3. An explanation of why Donna now requires insulin
      4. A demonstration of how to draw up and administer insulin
      5. Time for Donna to practice the skill on an orange
      6. Self-administration of insulin with Becky's guidance
      7. Time for questions and feedback
      8. A summary of the highlights of the lesson
      9. Handouts on diabetes and insulin administration for further reading
    10. Documentation of teaching on the client care record

V. *Evaluation:* On the next visit to Donna's room, Becky monitors Donna as she self-administers insulin. Following the injection, Becky validates Donna's success at learning the skill by completing the following checklist:

   ____ Washes hand before beginning procedure
   ____ Correctly identifies type of insulin and amount to be given
   ____ Selects correct syringe for insulin administration
   ____ Injects air equal to amount of medication to be given into insulin
   ____ Withdraws correct amount of insulin to be given
   ____ Removes all air bubbles from syringe and medication
   ____ Uses site rotation method to choose site for insulin administration
   ____ Cleanses site with alcohol and injects medication at SQ angle
   ____ Uses aseptic technique throughout entire procedure
   ____ Disposes of sharps in appropriate container
   ____ Washes hands and stores supplies properly

Next, she evaluates Donna's understanding of diabetes and self-care by asking questions about the lesson content. Each day, Donna and Becky discuss the three expected outcomes to see if they have been met. If not, changes will be planned to help Donna meet these goals before discharge home.

This sample case study illustrates the importance of ensuring that client teaching is indeed client-centered. As a registered nurse, you must accept client teaching as an integral part of your work (Hansen and Fisher, 1998). Regardless of whether or not you think of yourself as a teacher, you will be viewed by clients as a resource on health-related matters, so you must be prepared to answer questions. Clients are being exposed to increasingly more complex procedures and treatments, and must be prepared to make informed decisions about care.

Although many nurses recognize the importance of the role of the nurse as client educator, they often have insufficient training in the principles and concepts discussed in this chapter (Noble, 1991). Regardless of educational background, the nurse who keeps an open mind about client education, who looks for those opportunities to share knowledge with clients, and who approaches client teaching with enthusiasm is indeed a valuable asset to the profession.

CRITICAL THINKING EXERCISES

1. Identify a learning need for an adult client with hypertension. Write an expected outcome for each of the three learning domains (cognitive, affective, and psychomotor) that would be included in a teaching plan for this client.

    _____

    _____

    _____

    _____

    _____

    _____

2. Apply the learning need from the previous question to a seven-year-old girl with hypertension. Explain developmental differences that would need to be incorporated into the client teaching plan.

    _____

    _____

    _____

    _____

    _____

3. You are assigned to do discharge teaching to a new mother who does not speak English. She indicates an interest in learning about breastfeeding. Describe nursing interventions that would be appropriate to the teaching plan for this client.

    _____

    _____

    _____

    _____

    _____

4. Early in this chapter you were asked to describe a situation in which you provided teaching to a client/family. Explain what you would do differently with this same client now that you have learned about adult learning principles and development of a client teaching plan.

_____

_____

_____

_____

_____

_____

REFERENCES

Bloom, B. (1956). *Taxonomy of educational objectives: The classification of educational goals.* New York: David McKay.

Hansen, M., and J. Fisher (1998). Patient-centered teaching from theory to practice. *American Journal of Nursing* 98(1):56–60.

Harrington, N., N. Smith, and W. Spratt (1996). *LPN to RN transitions.* Philadelphia: Lippincott-Raven.

Hill, S., and H. Howlett (2001). *Success in practical nursing* (4th ed.). Philadelphia: W.B. Saunders.

Knowles, M. (1984). *The modern practice of adult education: From pedagogy to andragogy.* Chicago: Follett.

Leahy, J., and P. Kizilay (1998). *Foundations of nursing practice: A nursing process approach.* Philadelphia: W.B. Saunders.

Noble, C. (1991). Are nurses good patient educators? *Journal of Advanced Nursing* 16:1185–1189.

Palmerini, J., and D. Jasovsky (1998). Patient education: A guide for success. *Nursing Management* 29(8):45–46.

Redman, B. (1997). *The process of patient education* (8th ed.). St. Louis: Mosby–Year Book.

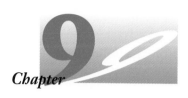

Chapter

Nursing Leadership and Management

LEARNING OBJECTIVES

After completing this chapter, you will be able to:

1. Discuss the differences between the leadership and management functions of registered nurses.
2. Apply various leadership theories to the management of health care personnel.
3. Analyze your own personality characteristics for strengths/weaknesses related to managing people.
4. Develop a unit-specific plan for managing conflict among staff, clients, and other health care personnel.
5. Discuss the role of the registered nurse in delegation of tasks to other personnel.
6. Discuss management strategies used to motivate staff to assist with planned change.
7. Describe the benefits of a case management approach to client care.

KEY TERMS

Authority

Case Manager

Change

Clinical Pathway

Conflict

Delegation

Front Line Management

Leadership

Leadership Styles

Autocratic

Democratic

Laissez Faire

Life-Cycle Theory

Management

Middle Management

Power

Top Level Management

Transformational
Leadership

 Maria, Kevin, and Suzanna are comparing grades on recently completed teaching projects.

Kevin: I'm really glad I got an A on my teaching project! But I have to tell you, it really caused me a problem at work when I tried to present it to my co-workers. They didn't like the idea of learning a new way to teach clients self-administration of insulin. They're very comfortable with the old way, and they don't seem willing to change.

Maria: I know what you mean. The people I work with have used the same forms for charting since I started there several years ago. I've tried to talk to our supervisor about revising our care plans—I've even offered to help her design them along a nursing process format. But she won't even discuss my ideas.

Suzanna: You both sound like the more you're learning, the more you want to teach your colleagues. But when you try sharing what you know, everyone just resents your suggestions. We're proud of our new knowledge, and we want to do a better job caring for clients. So why can't others just open their minds instead of feeling threatened? I believe that as we learn more in this program, we have a tendency to want to assume a leadership role in planning change. What's wrong with that? As future registered nurses, we're *supposed* to take responsibility for improving client care!

In recent years, a rapidly changing health care industry has shifted the focus of client care from the institution to the community. As nurses broaden the scope and setting of nursing practice, they assume greater independence and responsibility than ever before. Nurses are experiencing an increasing amount of pressure to advocate for clients, coordinate care, and cut health care costs.

Since the days of Florence Nightingale, nurses have led, directed, and organized client care. A vital link between the client and the health care system, nurses have become responsible for outcome management, team coordination, and continuity of care (Krejci and Malin, 1997). As nursing responsibilities increase, so does the need for effective leadership skills.

By becoming a registered nurse, you will assume more accountability for client care and the actions of other personnel than you had as an LPN/LVN. Even though nurses at all levels manage client care, the registered nurse controls decisions regarding staff and care of clients (Hill and Howlett, 2001). Practical/vocational nurses may be placed in charge nurse positions in some agencies, such as extended care facilities; however, the nurse manager (registered nurse) retains ultimate accountability for all nursing care activities.

The thought of managing other personnel is often intimidating to beginning nurses, perhaps because management theory and skills are not given as much instructional time as client care content in nursing programs. The purpose of this chapter is to build on management/leadership content you may have already had, present various theories on managing people, describe characteristics of effective managers, and discuss such management concerns as delegation, conflict resolution, and staff motivation. A multidisciplinary case management approach to client care will be explored as a part of the nurse's role as a manager of care.

LEADERSHIP AND MANAGEMENT: ARE THEY THE SAME?

The terms *leadership* and *management*, although sometimes used interchangeably, are actually separate . . . and quite distinct. **Leadership** is the ability to influence others in a manner that will get the job done. A leadership role is not an appointed position, but one given to the leader by a group of workers. According to Loveridge and Cummings (1996), leadership implies the use of creative thinking, excellent communication skills, and the will to act.

The leader must be able to guide others to accomplish desired tasks. Leaders acquire respect and authority from workers because they have demonstrated knowledge and skills and because they have the ability to make sound decisions. Frequently, nursing units possess *informal leaders*—people who have no appointed position of authority, but to whom others listen and lend support. Florence Nightingale is an excellent example of a leader, for she influenced others to bring about needed changes in health care in the British military services (see chapter 3).

Management consists of planning, organizing, directing, coordinating, and controlling activities designed to meet organizational goals (Marriner-Tomey, 2000). A manager is appointed to the position in the organization, and is accountable for effective use of available resources. In other words, a manager must manage both human and financial aspects of an organization. Responsibilities of a manager include the ability to assess situations in a rational manner, set unit goals, direct activities, maintain acceptable productivity, and monitor employee satisfaction (Loveridge and Cummings, 1996). An example of a manager is a nurse hired into the position of nurse manager, as he or she has the responsibility of managing and directing staff and client care activities.

Is it possible to be both a leader and a manager? Of course it is, and it is hoped that managers are also good leaders. Unfortunately, this is not always the case. When a nurse is placed in a management position, leadership authority does not automatically accompany the appointment. A manager must display effective leadership qualities to the staff in order to be able to motivate them to work toward unit objectives. By identifying and using informal leaders in a positive manner, a manager is better able to efficiently guide others toward goal accomplishment.

LEADERSHIP THEORIES AND MANAGEMENT STYLES

Several leadership and management theories exist and are used in practice to guide the development of each person's particular management style. One of the most commonly utilized leadership theories is that of Kurt Lewin (1947), who described three leadership styles: autocratic, democratic, and laissez faire. Figure 9–1 depicts the three styles on a continuum, ranging from greater control (autocratic) to less control (laissez faire) of employees.

In the autocratic style, the leader makes all decisions and allows no input from the workers. More emphasis is placed on task accomplishment than on concern for people. The authoritarian leader motivates others by coercion, and maintains strong control over the workers. This style tends to bring about dissatisfaction and loss of motivation in workers, which may eventually lead to

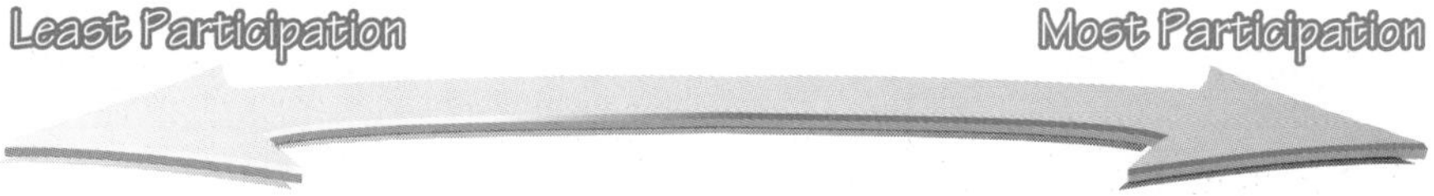

Least Participation   Most Participation

AUTOCRATIC	DEMOCRATIC	LAISSEZ FAIRE
Leader centered; controlled worker input	Worker centered; all workers have input; leader guides	Worker directed and controlled; no leader input
Efficient/rapid process (effective for quick decisions)	Time consuming process (effective for decision when worker satisfaction is desired)	Disorganized; time consuming (effective when innovative approach is desired)
Task oriented	Worker/process oriented	Task oriented
Nonparticipation decreases job satisfaction and motivation	Participation increases job satisfaction	Undirected participation increases frustration and decreases productivity

Figure 9–1
Leadership styles.

decreased productivity. There are, however, client situations that respond best to autocratic leadership. The following scenario is an example:

> Martha, Juan, and Samantha are new graduate nurses who are being oriented to work in a thoracic ICU. During the third week of their orientation, a client experiences a cardiopulmonary arrest. The unit nurse manager, who has not been involved in actual client care, arrives in the unit and begins to assign staff to specific tasks during the code. The three new graduates are instructed by the nurse manager to provide care to the unit's other clients, thereby allowing more experienced nurses to participate in the resuscitation efforts. Martha, Juan, and Samantha express concern afterwards to their preceptors about not being given the choice to view the resuscitation in order to gain experience.

What are your thoughts about the nurse manager's actions? Should the new graduates have been given the choice of watching the code? Explain your answer.

_____

_____

_____

_____

_____

_____

The **democratic** leader involves workers in decision making. Human relations and teamwork are important issues to the leader, who directs by suggestions and guidance. Communication is open between the leader and the staff. Workers who take part in this type of participative management report greater job satisfaction and group cohesiveness (Loveridge and Cummings, 1996). It must be emphasized, however, that this particular type of leader must be able to maintain final control of important decisions concerning client care and unit operation. Consider the following scenario:

> Melissa and Joe are nurses working on a psychiatric unit in a large teaching hospital that is planning to convert to a computerized system of charting. Both Melissa and Joe have expressed concern to the nurse manager regarding the use of the new system on their unit. Sensing their reluctance to learn a new system, the nurse manager assigns Melissa and Joe to represent the psychiatric unit on the hospital's task force that is selecting the new equipment.

Did the nurse manager make a wise decision in choosing Melissa and Joe to participate on the task force? Explain your answer. Do you believe their involvement will have a positive or negative influence on selection of a new system?

_____

_____

_____

_____

_____

Laissez faire, or free-rein, leadership refers to the complete autonomy of workers to make decisions without input from the group leader. If consulted, the leader provides assistance and guidance; however, the group is basically allowed to function independently of the leader. There is little or no control exerted over workers by the leader. This type of leadership style may, however, cause workers to feel a lack of feedback and direction. In settings where nurses function very autonomously (such as intensive care units and obstetrics), this style is popular, for it encourages independent decision making. The following is an example of laissez faire leadership:

> Henry and Sylvia are nurses who work on a pediatric unit. Their manager has been doing the nursing staff schedule on a monthly basis for many years. One afternoon during a staff meeting, the manager explains that he has decided to allow the nursing staff to schedule themselves. He will supply the form, fill in the needed shifts for each day, and ask the staff to negotiate among themselves for shifts, days off, and so forth.

What is your opinion of the nurse manager's decision? Do you believe the staff have been given too much control? Explain your opinion.

_____

_____

_____

_____

_____

Do any of the preceding leadership styles appear to be universally applicable in every management interaction with people? Generally, managers tend to use one of the three more often than the others, but apply the style that best fits each situation. For example, a manager who believes in a democratic form of leadership might use a laissez faire approach to allow staff to choose new uniforms for the unit personnel.

A second approach to leadership style, the life-cycle theory, was developed by Hersey and Blanchard. This approach suggests that leadership style may be determined by the level of maturity or immaturity of the followers (Hersey, 1984). *Maturity* is described as the level of security and competence each individual feels about the task to be completed. The leader assesses the worker's ability to complete the assigned task, and provides the appropriate leadership behavior that best meets the needs of the worker. Less mature personnel would require more delegation and direct supervision, while more mature individuals might be capable of participating in decision making regarding goal setting and task accomplishment. The maturity level of the group also helps determine how the leader communicates with them. The following examples show adaptation of leadership behavior according to group maturity:

> Emily is the nurse manager of an outpatient surgical unit in a small community hospital. The nurses on her unit have been together since the unit opened twelve years ago. They function very independently and rarely require assistance when presented with a client care problem. As a result, Emily allows them to help make most of the decisions regarding unit policies and goals.
>
> Brooke, manager of the post-anesthesia care unit in the same hospital, has a staff composed of relatively young nurses, most with less than three years' experience. Actively involved in day-to-day client care activities with the staff, Brooke is available to answer questions and assist with decision making. Unit policies and goals are primarily written by Brooke, with input from the nursing staff.

In 1985, Bennis and Nanus offered an approach to leadership that described four "human handling skills" common to leaders. The first skill, *attention through vision*, refers to the leader's ability to form a clear picture of outcomes for followers. *Meaning through communication*, the second skill, means the leader is able to convert the vision into images that others can understand through effective communication techniques. A third skill, *trust through positioning*, is the ability of the leader to inspire trust in others by taking the organization in the right direction. The leader maintains a constant position through both good and bad times. Finally, the fourth skill, *deployment of self through positive self-regard*, refers to the personal relationship that the leader cultivates with followers. Emphasizing positive personal strengths and compensating for weaknesses, the leader displays a positive self-image to followers.

An important component of this theory is that attitudes influence outcomes. A positive attitude that concentrates on success is a focus of this leadership style.

This theory, called **transformational leadership,** contends that such leaders empower their followers to action by allowing them to share in decision making (Bennis and Nanus, 1985). The transformational leader focuses on rewarding quality and excellence, rather than on punishing and manipulating to achieve outcomes.

Each manager must develop her own particular method of leading and managing others. This brief discussion of three different leadership theories will perhaps provide you with the groundwork upon which to build your own personal management style. Leadership skills do not come as naturally to some people as others, but can be learned and enhanced with education and experience.

THE EFFECTIVE NURSE MANAGER

In nursing, management occurs at all levels, from the bedside to the facility's administrative offices. Although managing people is different from managing client care, today's nurse must be adept at both; even bedside staff nurses are assuming more supervisory responsibilities because of the current trends of power decentralization and participatory management (Swansburg, 1996).

Health care organizations are generally divided into three levels of management: top, middle, and front line (Figure 9–2). **Top level management** is made

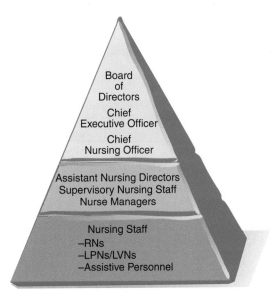

Figure 9–2
Levels of management.

up of the board of directors, the chief executive officer, and vice presidents of the organization. The chief nursing officer usually has a position at this level. **Middle level management** includes assistant directors of nursing and supervisory staff. Nurse managers occupy this level, directly overseeing nursing staff, who make up the third level, the **front line management** staff.

The higher the manager is in this hierarchy, the smaller the amount of client contact. Managers at the executive level primarily oversee organizational fiscal management, strategic planning, and coordination of care services (Swansburg, 1996). Middle managers supervise personnel of the front line level and are usually responsible for budgetary, staffing, and quality-care issues. Front line managers have the greatest client contact, managing client care while supervising nursing and ancillary personnel. Your first experience in managing people will probably be as a front line manager, acting as a team leader to oversee other nursing staff. You will answer to a unit nurse manager. Following is a partial list of the nurse manager's more common responsibilities:

1. Financial management of the unit
2. Hiring and staffing
3. Disciplinary action
4. Performance appraisals
5. Setting unit goals
6. Serving as role model and mentor
7. Coordinating professional development of the staff
8. Developing standards of care
9. Delegation of tasks to various personnel

As previously discussed, a manager is not necessarily a leader; but in order to be more effective as a manager, it is important to be a leader as well. The preceding list of duties describes tasks that are frequently performed by unit managers. But what about the more personal aspects of managing people—the ones emphasized in the previous section on management styles?

What personality characteristics do you believe are important in a leader/manager?

_____

_____

_____

_____

_____

_____

Which of these do you believe you possess? Which can be developed?

_____

_____

_____

_____

_____

_____

Examples of desirable leadership characteristics are listed in Box 9–1.

In addition, it is essential that managers possess the ability to think critically, make decisions under pressure, and bring about change through an orderly process. Nurse managers must be adept at managing human, financial, and informational resources in order to be effective (Craven and Hirnle, 2000).

THE NURSE AS A MANAGER OF PEOPLE

You thought you went into nursing to care for clients, not manage people, right? But someone must be responsible for supervising personnel who directly care for clients. And who is better suited to manage nurses than other nurses? Do you want a non-nurse telling you how to perform nursing duties?

As a manager of people, you may confront some of the following issues: authority vs. power, delegation, conflict, and change. The following sections briefly describe each concept and how they relate to nursing management.

Box 9-1   *Leadership Characteristics*

- Sound judgment
- Effective interpersonal skills
- Moral conscience
- Sense of fairness
- Adaptability
- Creativity
- Respect for others
- Self-confidence
- Ability to problem solve
- Effective stress management
- Commitment to continued personal growth

Authority vs. Power

The right to act in situations in which one is held accountable is called **authority** (Singer, 1997). An organization gives a manager official power, or authority, for certain actions, such as hiring, firing, and discipline. Managerial authority is necessary to maintain order in the work environment. Workers usually expect managers to exercise a given amount of authority, but may become resistant if they perceive too much control over their actions. An autocratic leader is an example of someone who may overuse the authority of her position.

Power, on the other hand, is the ability to influence others to do something they would not normally do (Marquis and Huston, 1999). For example, a nurse manager of an ICU has the authority to assign staff to care for specific clients. She may not, however, have the power to influence the staff to attend optional inservice classes. To be an effective manager, she must be perceived as having a certain amount of power over the nursing staff so they are willing to work with her on achieving unit goals.

French and Raven (1959) identified five sources of power:

1. legitimate
2. reward
3. coercive
4. expert
5. referent

A position of authority brings with it *legitimate power*, or the duty to command. *Reward power* is obtained from having the ability to grant favors. For example, a manager may use this type of power to give a staff member a day off in return for working overtime. *Coercive power* is the opposite of reward power. A manager may exercise this type of power by threatening unpleasant consequences for actions. A nurse who frequently arrives for work late may fear disciplinary action by the manager, who is exercising coercive power over the individual. *Expert power* is attained by demonstrating knowledge and/or skill expertise in a particular area. Staff nurses may look to a manager for guidance and direction because of clinical expertise. Finally, when the staff perceive a manager to be powerful because of personal characteristics such as charisma, that manager is said to exhibit *referent power*. Certain people are viewed as powerful simply because others agree with their beliefs and what they symbolize (Marquis and Huston, 1999).

Nurse managers need to recognize how to effectively use authority and power to motivate others to accomplish tasks and bring about needed change. By judiciously utilizing authority, managers can prevent resentment in employees. An understanding of appropriate uses of power will guide a manager's actions in ways that foster staff cooperation. Managers who empower their followers are themselves empowered.

Delegation

It is impossible for one person to perform all the client care activities required in a day, so nurses must delegate part of their tasks to others. Whether you are in a formal management position or are functioning as a staff nurse on a client care unit, delegation is a necessity.

The National Council of State Boards of Nursing (1990) defines delegation as "entrusting the performance of selected nursing tasks to competent persons in selected situations. The nurse retains the accountability for the total nursing care of the individuals." This definition implies two things:

1. The person to whom the task is delegated must be competent to perform it.
2. The nurse is still responsible for ensuring the job is done right.

Note: It is important to point out that the delegate for the task is accountable for her own actions.

A common misconception of the beginning nurse is that she must be a "super-nurse" and juggle a large number of tasks alone. Fortunately, delegation makes it possible for nurses to assign some duties to other capable personnel while *still retaining accountability for the client care.* The following guidelines will assist you in knowing how and when to delegate:

1. Assess the workload to determine what can be delegated
2. Identify the skill level necessary to complete the job effectively
3. Choose the person best able to do the job (Table 9–1)
4. Give clear directions and make sure the task is fully understood
5. Obtain an agreement to do the job
6. Set a sufficient amount of time for job completion
7. Make sure necessary equipment is available
8. Offer assistance if needed and monitor progress
9. Follow up on completion and give appropriate feedback

TABLE 9–1
Resources for Choosing the Best Candidate for Task Delegation

RESOURCE	INFORMATION PROVIDED
Employee job descriptions	Employee skills and job expectations
Policies and procedures	Who may perform skills and how
Staffing schedule	Number of personnel on unit and their job titles
Unit census	Number of clients on unit; other pertinent information
Employee skills/competencies	Skills personnel proficient at performing and dates of check-off
State Nurse Practice Act	Scope of nursing; what may be delegated and to whom

Delegation issues are not always easy to resolve. Consider the following scenario, which takes place on a busy surgical unit:

> Wendy, the evening charge nurse, is responsible for managing a nursing staff of three other nurses and two nursing assistants. The unit census is currently 24 clients, most of whom have had surgery one to two days previously. From information received during shift change report, Wendy is especially concerned about Blake Andrew, a young man who has a new tracheostomy. The day-shift nurses reported that Blake has complained of difficulty breathing since returning from surgery. Wendy must assign one of the following nurses to care for Blake:
>
> Abby—a new graduate with three months' experience
> Matt—four years of experience, two of which were in ICU
> Adam—nine years of experience, the majority in long-term care

What factors should enter into Wendy's decision?

_____

_____

_____

_____

_____

_____

Should she consider years and type of nursing experience? What about choosing Abby, who has recent knowledge of tracheostomy care from nursing school? Or should she delegate to Matt, who has experience with unstable clients? Adam has worked in long-term care, which may have given him tracheostomy care experience; but does he have the judgment and assessment skills to care for a potentially critical client? At first glance, it would appear that Matt would probably be the best candidate for caring for a client who needs close monitoring. Wendy's decision should be based on each individual nurse's skills and ability to care for the client, as well as other factors, such as acuity level of other clients on the unit.

Never assume a person is capable of doing a delegated task simply because her job description says she can. For instance, an agency may allow nursing assistants to insert indwelling urinary catheters; however, training programs vary, so many nursing assistants may not know this skill. By communicating with the person about her qualifications before assigning a task, you may avoid problems.

The National Council of State Boards of Nursing (1990) recommends a decision making process for delegation which also addresses the potential for harm, the frequency with which the delegate has performed the task, and the client's ability for input into the choice of caregiver. By gathering as much information as possible before delegating, nurses demonstrate leadership skills and decrease the potential for error (Fisher, 1999).

Do not forget to use good assessment skills and professional judgment when delegating portions of nursing care to others. Remember, the client's best interests should be the guiding criteria by which you make decisions regarding delegation of care.

Conflict

Internal discord resulting from differing opinions between two or more people, or **conflict,** can be a source of great job stress (Marquis and Huston, 1999). In a health care setting, conflict may occur because of competition between individuals or departments over resources, because individuals disagree about a course of action, or because the fast-paced environment sets the stage for differences. Disagreements take place between nurses, peers, physicians, clients, and other health care workers.

The effective nurse manager must be knowledgeable about conflict resolution techniques (discussed in more detail in chapter 5) in order to maintain a harmonious working environment. According to Arnold and Boggs (1999), there are four personal styles of conflict management:

1. avoidance
2. accommodation
3. competition
4. collaboration

Perhaps the most often used strategy for managing conflict is the passive one of avoidance. When a situation generates feelings of intense discomfort, many people tend to withdraw, rather than face the issue head on. Unfortunately, avoiding an issue that has not been resolved does not accomplish closure. The manager who avoids dealing with a problem employee only prolongs the inevitable, and often makes a bad situation worse.

Accommodation is another passive means of dealing with conflict. The accommodating manager cooperates or gives false reassurances instead of dealing with the issue. Such attempts to maintain peace only defer the problem, avoiding confrontation until a later time. For example, when a manager gives in to an angry staff member's demands for a day off when the unit is already short-staffed, the stage is set for future similar demands.

Competition is a style of conflict management consisting of domination of one person over the other. Generally, one person is the aggressor, demanding her own way, regardless of the consequences to others. The dictatorial manager may employ this technique to gain control over employees in times of conflict.

During collaboration, both parties agree to work together to find a mutually satisfying solution to the conflict. Considered to be the most effective style for actually resolving conflict, this method directly confronts the issue. Both sides of the problem are addressed, and steps are taken to work collaboratively to ensure a positive outcome for both sides.

Which of the four conflict management styles described best fits the way you deal with personal conflict? Explain:

_____

_____

_____

_____

_____

_____

Before becoming effective at resolving conflict, you must first understand your personal style of conflict management. Avoidance and accommodating behaviors may encourage the staff to like you. But are you striving to make friends or to be a good manager? A competitive attitude may temporarily bring about order during chaos; but if it is utilized frequently, the competitive approach will cause a stressful, tense work atmosphere.

Practice assertive behavior instead of reacting emotionally and aggressively to conflict. Encourage all involved to look carefully at both sides of a problem and to work together toward a solution. An important aspect of managing people is the ability to guide them in working together to formulate solutions to problems.

Change

Human beings are largely creatures of habit; however, **change** is inevitable, especially in the workplace. Nurses in leadership positions are expected to implement organizational change, which involves motivating personnel to become a part of new ways of doing things (Figure 9–3).

When confronted with change, people usually react by either *resisting* or *assisting*. By reacting negatively and refusing to take part in change, people miss out on the opportunity to give input. Therefore, if they remain within the organization, they are forced to do things according to the decisions of others.

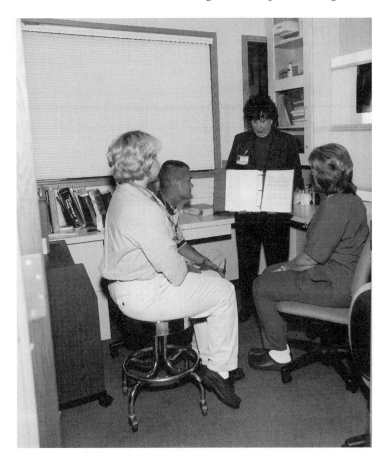

Figure 9-3
Nurse managers implement change by involving staff members.

As change occurs, they may experience discomfort and feelings of being over-whelmed in a previously comfortable, familiar environment.

Marquis and Huston (1999) list four rules for nurse managers to remember when implementing change:

1. Change should be implemented only for a good reason, such as to solve a problem or improve work efficiency.
2. Resistance to change is natural and should be anticipated.
3. Change should be planned, when possible, and implemented gradually.
4. Those affected by change should be involved in the planning and imple-mentation.

Kurt Lewin (1951) identified three stages that must be experienced before change is integrated into the organization:

1. unfreezing
2. movement
3. refreezing

During *unfreezing*, the status quo is questioned, and the person begins to feel that change is needed. The situation is analyzed to determine if change is possible; others may be polled about their feelings and sometimes may be influenced to believe that change is needed. The picture of the way things have been is beginning to change.

The *movement* stage of change involves setting goals and developing strategies to bring about the proposed change. An analysis of supporting and resisting factors is done in order to determine if change is possible at this time. Actions are taken to implement the change, and evaluation is done. A new picture is being formed from the old, and is taking a new shape.

Refreezing consists of continuing to monitor outcomes of the change and supporting efforts to sustain the effects. This includes evaluating the impact on people and services and making necessary revisions to maintain the desired outcomes. The new picture is now in the employees' minds, with shapes from the old incorporated within.

But what about those staff who do not want to change? What strategies are available to the manager who is attempting to motivate others to move together in a positive direction that will bring about needed change? The following are suggestions for handling barriers to change:

- Talk with staff to discover the basis for resistance.
- Dispel any unfounded ideas about negative outcomes.
- Present more positive information about proposed outcomes.
- Form a task force to work on possible ways to implement the change, including staff who resist the plan.
- Discuss the proposed change as "our" plan rather than "my" plan.
- Be persistent in trying to win over staff.
- Be open to suggested alterations to the original plan for change.
- Work with staff to find the easiest way to implement the planned change.

The wise manager understands underlying reasons for resistance to change among staff members. For example, an older employee may worry about not being able to learn a new system, such as computerized laboratory requests. It is critical that managers find effective methods for helping all staff members adjust to change in ways that will allow them to maintain a healthy sense of self-esteem.

Havelock (1973), in writing about change theory, described a *change agent* as a person who facilitates planned change. Change agents set the stage for change, facilitate the process, and trouble-shoot when there are problems. Nurses at all levels in an organization can function as change agents, from the client bedside to the administrative offices. By being part of the change process, nurses ensure their input into decisions that will ultimately affect client care outcomes.

Perhaps this discussion on common problem areas in managing people has left you nervous about assuming a management role. Conflicts, power struggles, and the need for change are facts of life, especially in the health care work environment, where stressors abound. By understanding strategies useful in dealing with such issues, the nurse manager will be better prepared to effectively lead other staff in achieving unit goals.

THE NURSE AS A MANAGER OF CARE

With the advent of DRGs (Diagnostic Related Groups) and managed care (see chapter 3), nursing care delivery systems have had to change to meet the demand for more accountability (Conger, 1999). The **case manager** role has evolved in nursing, defined as a process of managing and coordinating health care services in a time- and cost-effective manner. Other disciplines, such as social work, have case-managed clients for years. More recently, nurses have become involved in coordination of services in all aspects of client care—the home, the outpatient clinic, the hospital, and the extended care facility.

Nursing case management is advantageous for several reasons. First, client care is coordinated across a continuum of health or illness, ensuring continuity of care. Second, quality care outcomes are monitored. Third, clients and families have greater access to personnel and services. Finally, the cost-effectiveness of tests and procedures is monitored (Williams-Lee, 1999).

When a client enters a health care system in which nursing case management is used, the nurse uses the nursing process to assess, diagnose, and develop expected outcomes. Many agencies then institute a **clinical pathway** that guides care toward achievement of expected outcomes (see Figure 9–4). A clinical pathway (also called a *critical pathway* or *care path*) is a multidisciplinary plan of care that outlines the optimal sequencing and timing of interventions for particular diagnoses, procedures, or symptoms (Ignatavicius and Hausman, 1995). Incorporated within the pathway are client teaching and discharge planning. When utilized, clinical pathways help keep staff "on track" with the plan of care in order to provide quality care, prevent complications, and decrease costs.

The nurse case manager may or may not have graduate level training; however, the case manager role requires high level nursing skills, the ability to manage people, and effective communication patterns. As a case manager, the nurse carries a caseload of clients who may be at any point within the health care system—at home, the hospital, in an extended care facility, and so forth. Throughout the process, the nurse coordinates care with other disciplines and

MISSOURI DELTA MEDICAL CENTER
Sikeston, Missouri

Clinical Path—Congestive Heart Failure
ANTICIPATED LOS: 4 DAYS

Problem #1: LEARNING NEEDS REGARDING MANAGEMENT OF CONGESTIVE HEART FAILURE

Nursing Diagnosis: **Knowledge Deficit**

Date Initiated ________ By: ______________ Date Resolved: ________ By: ______________

Expected Outcome
1. Patient will verbalize understanding of management of respiratory function, diet, monitoring of fluid/weight, activity, and medications.

Nursing Assessment/ Interventions (Practice Standards)
1. Assess Patient's/Family's current knowledge.
2. Evaluate if Patient/Family can verbalize/demonstrate information taught.
3. Provide individualized instruction on specific aspect of care.
4. Review, reinforce, and modify teaching methods as needed.
5. Implement Patient Path, give handouts.

Problem #2: CARDIAC INSUFFICIENCY

Nursing Diagnosis: **Decreased Cardiac Output**

Date Initiated: ________ By: ______________ Date Resolved: ________ By: ______________

Expected Outcome:
1. Patient's heart rate and rhythm will be within normal limits for patient.

Nursing Assessment/ Interventions (Practice Standards)
1. Assess for respiratory rate > 20, SOB, use of accessory muscles, lung sounds, heart tones, Dysrhythmias, cyanosis, diaphoresis, edema, intake and output, daily weight
2. Assist patient to Cardiac Position (HOB and knees up) to aid respiratory effort
3. Administer medications as ordered
4. Administer O_2 at 2 L per nasal cannula.

Problem #3: ______________________________

Nursing Diagnosis: ______________________________

Date Initiated ________ By: ______________ Date Resolved: ________ By: ______________

Expected Outcome:
1. ______________________________

Nursing Assessment/ Interventions (Practice Standards)
1. ______________________________
2. ______________________________
3. ______________________________
4. ______________________________
5. ______________________________

☐ PATIENT PATH EDUCATION INFORMATION GIVEN TO **AND** REVIEWED WITH PATIENT AND/OR FAMILY.

Date Patient Pathway Reviewed: ________ By: ______________

The suggested plan represents the initial desired course of treatment and goals of recovery. These are average guidelines only and should be reviewed periodically by the attending physician and other involved disciplines. Deviations are generally expected and revisions to the plan should be made as warranted.

Form CP 7 C   Orig: 5/98, Rev: 6/98, 6/00

Figure 9–4
Clinical Pathway (Used with permission from Missouri Delta Medical Center.)

MISSOURI DELTA MEDICAL CENTER
Sikeston, Mo.

Congestive Heart Failure Clinical Pathway
ALOS = 4 DAYS

CARE GIVER'S INITIALS →	DATE: _____ DAY 4 D _____ E _____ N _____	DATE: _____ DAY 4 EXPECTED OUTCOMES	DISCHARGED BY:_____ TIME: _____
ASSESS-MENT	☐ Daily weight ☐ ☐ ☐ Monitor ☐ ☐ ☐ I & O q 8 hours ☐ ☐ ☐ * Chest Pain ___ ___ ___ HR < 120 ___ ___ ___ Resp rate < 30 ___ ___ ___ Skin intact	_____ Voices understanding weighing daily and recording _____ Heart rate WNL for patient _____ Respiratory rate WNL for patient _____ Lung sounds WNL for patient _____ I & O adequate for patient _____ Skin remains intact without redness or edema	
CONSULTS		_____ Voices understanding discharge plans	
TESTS/LABS		_____ Voices understanding follow-up appointment	
MEDS	☐ ☐ ☐ Heparin Lock ☐ ☐ ☐ O₂ ☐ ☐ ☐ Tylenol PRN ☐ ☐ ☐ Phenergan PRN ☐ ☐ ☐ Restoril PRN ☐ ☐ ☐ NTG PRN ___ ___ ___ Voices pain control	_____ Voices understanding medications and regimen _____ Remains pain free	
MOBILITY ADLs	☐ ☐ ☐ As tolerated ___ ___ ___ Tolerated w/out pain	_____ Tolerates ADL's without pain or SOB	
NUTRITION	☐ ☐ ☐ No added salt diet ☐ ☐ ☐ 2000cc daily fluid restriction	_____ Voices understanding low salt diet _____ Voices understanding 2000cc fluid restriction	
ELIMINA-TION	☐ ☐ ☐ Foley ___ ___ ___ UOP > 240cc in 8 hrs	_____ I & O WNL for patient	
TEACHING/ DC PLANNING	☐ ☐ ☐ Review home instructions ___ ___ ___ Uses pain scale ___ ___ ___ States S/S CHF ___ ___ ___ Complies w/2000cc Fluid Restriction ___ ___ ___ Complies with Low Salt Diet ___ ___ ___ Voices Understanding	☐ ☐ ☐ Review home instructions ___ ___ ___ Uses pain scale ___ ___ ___ States S/S CHF ___ ___ ___ Complies w/2000cc Fluid Restriction ___ ___ ___ Complies with Low Salt Diet ___ ___ ___ Voices Understanding CHF protocol and interventions	

SYMBOL KEY: ☐ = INTERVENTIONS
("I" STATEMENTS)

___ = EXPECTED OUTCOMES
("E" STATEMENTS)

✔ in box = intervention or item completed
0 in box = item not pertinent to your shift
+ in box = item not done on your shift
* in box = elaborate in nurses notes

PAIN SCALE

|_|_|_|_|_|_|_|_|_|_|
1   2   3   4   5   6   7   8   9   10

NO PAIN   MODERATE   WORSE

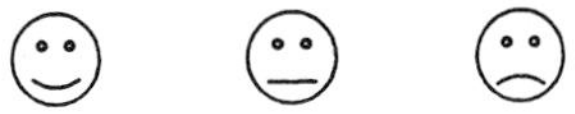

SIGNATURES: _____ _____ _____

FORM CP 7F   Orig: 5/98, Rev: 6/98, 3/00

Figure 9–4
Continued

Illustration continued on following page

Congestive Heart Failure Clinical Pathway
ALOS = 4 DAYS

CARE GIVER'S INITIALS →	DATE: _____ DAY 1 D ____ E ____ N ____	DATE: _____ DAY 2 D ____ E ____ N ____	DATE: _____ DAY 3 D ____ E ____ N ____
ASSESS-MENT	☐ ☐ ☐ Wt on Admission ☐ ☐ ☐ Monitor ☐ ☐ ☐ ☐ I & O q 8 hours ☐ ☐ ☐ * Chest Pain ___ ___ ___ HR < 120 ___ ___ ___ Resp rate < 30 ___ ___ ___ Skin intact	☐ Daily weight ☐ ☐ ☐ Monitor ☐ ☐ ☐ I & O q 8 hours ☐ ☐ ☐ * Chest Pain ___ ___ ___ HR < 120 ___ ___ ___ Resp rate < 30 ___ ___ ___ Skin intact	☐ Daily weight ☐ ☐ ☐ Monitor ☐ ☐ ☐ I & O q 8 hours ☐ ☐ ☐ * Chest Pain ___ ___ ___ HR < 120 ___ ___ ___ Resp rate < 30 ___ ___ ___ Skin intact
CONSULTS	☐ ☐ ☐ Internal Med/Cardio ☐ ☐ ☐ Dietitian ☐ ☐ ☐ Discharge Planner		
TESTS/LABS	**Results Assessed:** ☐ ☐ ☐ CXR ☐ ☐ ☐ EKG ☐ ☐ ☐ CPK & MB q 8 hr ☐ ☐ ☐ Chem 7, Mag, PT, PTT ☐ ☐ ☐ Dig level if applicable ☐ ☐ ☐ Pulse Ox ☐ ☐ ☐ ABG if P Ox < 92% ___ ___ ___ Dr aware of Abnorms	**Results Assessed:** ☐ ☐ ☐ EKG ☐ ☐ ☐ Chem 7, Magnesium ☐ ☐ ☐ Pulse Ox ☐ ☐ ☐ ABG if P Ox < 92% ___ ___ ___ Dr aware of Abnorms	☐ ☐ ☐ No added salt diet ☐ ☐ ☐ 2000cc daily fluid restriction
MEDS	☐ ☐ ☐ Heparin Lock ☐ ☐ ☐ O₂ ☐ ☐ ☐ Tylenol PRN ☐ ☐ ☐ Phenergan PRN ☐ ☐ ☐ Restoril PRN ☐ ☐ ☐ NTG PRN ___ ___ ___ Voices pain control	☐ ☐ ☐ Heparin Lock ☐ ☐ ☐ O₂ ☐ ☐ ☐ Tylenol PRN ☐ ☐ ☐ Phenergan PRN ☐ ☐ ☐ Restoril PRN ☐ ☐ ☐ NTG PRN ___ ___ ___ Voices pain control	☐ ☐ ☐ Heparin Lock ☐ ☐ ☐ O₂ ☐ ☐ ☐ Tylenol PRN ☐ ☐ ☐ Phenergan PRN ☐ ☐ ☐ Restoril PRN ☐ ☐ ☐ NTG PRN ___ ___ ___ Voices pain control
MOBILITY ADLs	☐ ☐ ☐ BR or BRP	☐ ☐ ☐ As tolerated ___ ___ ___ Tolerates w/out pain	☐ ☐ ☐ As tolerated ___ ___ ___ Tolerates w/out pain
NUTRITION	☐ ☐ ☐ No added salt diet ☐ ☐ ☐ 2000cc daily fluid restriction	☐ ☐ ☐ No added salt diet ☐ ☐ ☐ 2000cc daily fluid restriction	☐ ☐ ☐ No added salt diet ☐ ☐ ☐ 2000cc daily fluid restriction
ELIMINA-TION	☐ ☐ ☐ Foley ___ ___ ___ UOP > 240cc in 8 hrs	☐ ☐ ☐ Foley ___ ___ ___ UOP > 240cc in 8 hrs	☐ ☐ ☐ Foley ___ ___ ___ UOP > 240cc in 8 hrs
TEACHING/ DC PLANNING	☐ ☐ ☐ Teach use of pain scale ☐ ☐ ☐ Received Pt/Fam Handout ☐ ☐ ☐ Review S/S CHF ☐ ☐ ☐ Review Fluid Restriction ☐ ☐ ☐ Review Low Salt Diet ___ ___ ___ Voices Understanding	☐ ☐ ☐ Review Home Instructions ☐ ☐ ☐ Review S/S CHF ☐ ☐ ☐ Review Fluid Restriction ☐ ☐ ☐ Review Low Salt Diet ___ ___ ___ Uses pain scale ___ ___ ___ Voices Understanding	☐ ☐ ☐ Review Home Instructions ___ ___ ___ Uses pain scale ___ ___ ___ States S/S CHF ___ ___ ___ Complies w/2000cc fld restriction ___ ___ ___ Complies with Low Salt Diet ___ ___ ___ Voices Understanding

SYMBOL KEY: ☐ = **INTERVENTIONS**   ___ = **EXPECTED OUTCOMES**
                    ("I" STATEMENTS)   ("E" STATEMENTS)

✔ in box = intervention or item completed
0 in box = item not pertinent to your shift
+ in box = item not done on your shift
● in box = elaborate in nurses notes

PAIN SCALE

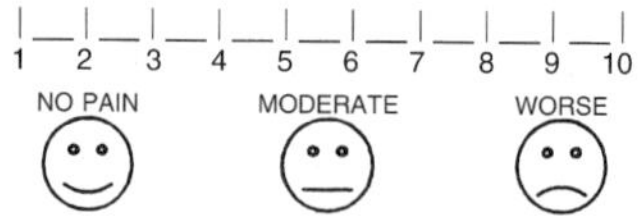

|_|_|_|_|_|_|_|_|_|_|
1 2 3 4 5 6 7 8 9 10
NO PAIN   MODERATE   WORSE

SIGNATURES: _____ _____

FORM CP 7E   Orig: 5/98, Rev: 6/98, 8/00

Figure 9-4
Continued

agencies and helps the client and family obtain needed supplies and other assistance. The ultimate goal is to assist the client to achieve expected outcomes, which include preventing further complications that would require hospitalization and increased health care costs.

Today's ever-changing health care environment requires that nurses be adept at coordinating care for groups of clients, managing other personnel, and keeping an eye turned toward cost containment. Knowledge of leadership and management theories, and of common pitfalls in dealing with people, will assist the nurse to survive in the work setting. The management of client care has taken on new meaning to nurses, since concerns over health care spending have threatened to dominate health care choices. Nurses must enter the work force prepared to use and refine both leadership and management skills.

CRITICAL THINKING EXERCISES

1. Compare and contrast the positive characteristics of autocratic, democratic, and laissez faire leadership styles.

_____

_____

_____

_____

_____

_____

2. You are a new graduate nurse on a surgical nursing unit. Today is your first day to be in charge of the unit. Describe how you would go about deciding which staff member to whom you would delegate the care of an unconscious stroke client. Other unit nursing staff consist of two experienced practical nurses, one experienced registered nurse, and two nursing assistants.

_____

_____

_____

_____

_____

_____

3. Consider a time when you have experienced conflict with another employee while at work. Utilizing a collaborative style of conflict management, list steps that could be used to resolve the problem.

_____

_____

_____

_____

_____

_____

4. Discuss at least three reasons why a nursing case management approach to client care is beneficial.

_____

_____

_____

_____

_____

REFERENCES

Arnold, E., and K. Boggs (1999). *Interpersonal relationships: Professional communication skills for nurses.* (3rd ed.). Philadelphia: W.B. Saunders.

Bennis, W., and B. Nanus (1985). *Leadership: The strategies for taking charge.* New York: Harper & Row.

Conger, M. (1999). *Managed care: Practice strategies for nursing.* Thousand Oaks, CA: Sage.

Craven, R., and C. Hirnle (2000). *Fundamentals of nursing: Human health and function* (3rd ed.). Philadelphia: Lippincott Williams & Wilkins.

Fisher, M. (1999). Do your nurses delegate effectively? *Nursing Management* 30(5):23–26.

French, J., and B. Raven (1959). The bases of social power. In *Studies in social power,* D. Cartwright, ed. Ann Arbor, MI: University of Michigan Press.

Havelock, R. (1973). *The change agent's guide to innovation in education.* Englewood Cliffs, NJ: Educational Technology Publications.

Hersey, P. (1984). *The situational leader.* New York: Warner Books.

Hill, S., and H. Howlett (2001). *Success in practical nursing: Personal and vocational issues* (4th ed.). Philadelphia: W.B. Saunders.

Ignatavicius, D., and K. Hausman (1995). *Clinical pathways for collaborative practice.* Philadelphia: W.B. Saunders.

Krejci, J., and S. Malin (1997). Impact of leadership development on competencies. *Nursing Economics* 15(5):235–241.

Lewin, K. (1947). Frontiers in group dynamics: Concept, method, and reality in social science, social equilibria, and social change. *Human Relations* 1(1):1–23.

Lewin, K. (1951). *Field theory in social sciences.* New York: Harper & Row.

Loveridge, C., and S. Cummings (1996). *Nursing management in the new paradigm.* Gaithersburg, MD: Aspen.

Marriner-Tomey, A. (2000). *Guide to nursing management and leadership* (6th ed.). St. Louis: Mosby/Harcourt Health Sciences.

Marquis, B., and C. Huston (1999). *Leadership roles and management functions in nursing: Theory and application* (3rd ed.). Philadelphia: J.B. Lippincott.

National Council of State Boards of Nursing (1990). Concept paper on delegation. Chicago.

Singer, C. (1997). Challenges of nursing management. In *Nursing today: Transition and trends* (2nd ed.), J. Zerwekh and J. Claborn, eds. Philadelphia: W.B. Saunders.

Swansburg, R. (1996). *Management and leadership for nurse managers* (2nd ed.). Boston: Jones & Bartlett.

Williams-Lee, P. (1999). Case management nips costs, not care. *Nursing Management* 30(10):12.

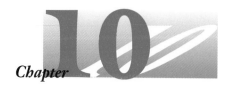

Chapter

Legal/Ethical Components of Nursing

LEARNING OBJECTIVES

After completing this chapter, you will be able to:

1. Discuss the importance of understanding how state nurse practice acts regulate professional nursing practice.
2. Incorporate legal principles of client care into daily nursing activities.
3. Develop a plan for implementing risk management measures into personal practice.
4. Analyze personal values to develop an understanding of their influence on clients during ethical decision making.
5. Identify conflicting ethical principles in ethically challenging client care situations.
6. Apply a personal framework for ethical decision making to client care.

KEY TERMS

Advance Directives	Ethical Dilemma	Nurse Practice Acts
ANA Code of Ethics	False Imprisonment	Patient Self-Determination Act
Assault	Fidelity	Risk Management
Autonomy	Incident Report	Statutory Laws
Battery	Informed Consent	Teleology
Beneficence	Justice	Values
Confidentiality	Malpractice	Veracity
Deontology	Nonmaleficence	

Maria, Kevin, and Suzanna are on a fifteen-minute break from their nursing theory class.

Kevin: You know, I don't think it'll be too hard for me to be a charge nurse on my shift when we finish this program. I've had plenty of experience helping the RN on our unit make decisions. It doesn't seem that difficult. I look forward to being in management someday.

Suzanna: Oh, I don't feel that way at all! I'm not comfortable telling other people what to do. I guess I'll need more experience as a nurse before I have the self-confidence to make assignments and give orders.

Maria: In my job in long-term care, I'm already in charge from time to time. It isn't too hard once you learn to organize your time and get used to being unpopular with the staff . . . especially when you make assignments they don't like. What's really frustrating is ethical problems. I hate it when I'm involved in an ethical dilemma with a resident or a family and the doctor. That's when I'm definitely not in control of the situation.

As client care becomes more complex and technological advances create new means to prolong life, nurses are being placed in the difficult position of not always knowing what is legally and ethically correct. Because they have such close contact with clients, nurses frequently find themselves in the role of client advocate when difficult decisions need to be made. Not only do nurses need to be able to assist clients through uncertain choices, they must also be assured that their actions do not place them at legal risk.

Legal/ethical issues of client care have long been of concern for nurses, who do not always feel as equipped to deal with such problems as with other day-to-day client needs. Fear of malpractice suits causes many nurses to be hesitant to care for disgruntled clients. The stress of ethical dilemmas in practice is a common factor related to low job satisfaction among nurses (Katims, 1998).

This chapter combines legal and ethical issues pertinent to nursing and client care, as they often overlap in actual practice. According to Hall (1996), "Law is a minimum standard of morality" (p. 2). As a registered nurse, you'll need a good understanding of laws and statutes governing your practice, and you'll have to know how to protect yourself from legal action.

Ethical decision making, often an emotional, stressful aspect of client care, can be approached more confidently with a basic understanding of values and ethics in nursing. The content presented here will provide the registered nurse with a foundation for safe, ethical nursing practice that incorporates a decision making framework into client care.

REGULATION OF NURSING PRACTICE

As you begin your journey down the road to becoming a registered nurse, it is essential that you become familiar with laws, agencies, and health care changes that will have a legal impact upon your practice. Federal, criminal, and civil laws, as well as state nurse practice acts and evolving bioethical/legal issues, are but a few of the factors influencing current nursing care of clients.

It is not possible for nurses to know all the laws that affect client care. However, nurses do need to be aware of the types of laws regulating their practice (Hall, 1996). **Statutory laws**—laws established through formal legislative processes (Betts and Waddle, 1997)—include *criminal* (unlawful behavior that threatens society) and *civil* laws (issues between individuals). Wrongs committed under criminal law are called *crimes*, whereas wrongs committed under civil statutes are called *torts*.

Each nurse must practice under statutory laws set forth by individual state legislatures; these state-mandated laws are known as **Nurse Practice Acts.** State Boards of Nursing have the responsibility of ensuring that the rules and regulations in their respective nurse practice acts are followed (Sheehan, 1997). Upon passing the licensure exam, the practical/vocational nurse or registered nurse must practice within the scope of the duties described in the nurse practice act in the state where she is licensed. Box 10–1 lists common elements of most state nurse practice acts. Once employed, the nurse is responsible for ensuring that the employing agency's job duties are congruent with those of the state's nurse practice act and other state and federal laws.

Various changes in health care have created legal issues for nurses that are still being explored. For example, with the increase in the number of advanced practice nurses (master's degree and above), prescriptive authority and autonomous prac-

Box 10-1   *Nurse Practice Acts*

- Define the scope of nursing practice in the state
- Control who may use nursing titles
- Outline educational requirements for entry into practice and licensure
- Identify causes for which disciplinary action may be taken against a licensee

tice are under debate in many states. Should nurse practitioners be allowed to prescribe controlled substances? Do they need to enter into a collaborative practice agreement with a physician? These are common questions, and they are generating much discussion among policy makers. Other concerns include issues related to delegation of client care to unlicensed assistive personnel (see chapter 9), reimbursement for services, and advance directives (discussed later in this chapter).

As a registered nurse, you can participate in shaping the laws that govern your practice. The American Nurses' Association (ANA) is one political voice for nurses, as are other nursing organizations. By joining such organizations and becoming active, you can contribute to legislative decisions affecting nursing. These organizations are working to ensure that nurses are allowed to participate in setting guidelines to regulate practice.

LEGAL ISSUES IN NURSING

Despite the difficulty of knowing every legal pitfall awaiting the nurse in the care of clients, it is important to understand the legal system, terminology, and commonly occurring problems. Table 10–1 contains a list of legal terms and definitions that are of importance in nursing. The following legal issues may arise as a result of nursing activities, intentional or not, and are a cause for concern.

Malpractice

Perhaps the greatest legal fear of each practicing nurse is that of being accused of nursing **malpractice**, or negligence in performing professional duties (Stark, 1997). Malpractice includes both acts of *omission* (not doing what should be done) and *commission* (doing what should not be done). When a nurse is charged with malpractice, she will be judged according to the prevailing standard of care, or what another reasonably prudent nurse would have done under the same circumstances.

For a plaintiff to show that a nurse is indeed guilty of malpractice, the following must be proven:

- The nurse had a duty to care for the client.
- The nurse breached the duty by failing to meet the standard of care.
- The client was harmed as a result of the breach of duty.
- A cause-and-effect relationship exists between the breach of duty and the injury.

TABLE 10-1
Common Legal Terms

TERMS	DEFINITIONS
Statutory laws	Laws passed through formal legislative processes
Torts	Civil wrongs committed against another person
Standard of care	What a reasonably prudent nurse would have done under similar circumstances
Good Samaritan laws	Laws enacted to protect health care workers who provide care in emergency situations
Expert witness	A person with expert knowledge and skills in a particular area
Defendant	The person who is accused of wrongdoing in a lawsuit
Malpractice	Failure to meet the standard of care in professional duties that results in harm to a person
Negligence	Failure to act as a reasonably prudent person would under similar circumstances
Reasonable care	The level of care or skill normally used by a competent health care worker of similar education and experience
Plaintiff	The person who claims harm or injury in a lawsuit; the one who files the suit
Libel	Defamation of a person's reputation by written word
Slander	Defamation of a person's reputation by spoken language

Nurses are expected to be competent to perform client care activities, and will be held accountable for failure to do so. Consider the following scenario:

Katie Leigh is a registered nurse working on a gynecology unit in a small town. She is frequently put in charge of the staff, which consists of one other RN and two nursing assistants. The unit usually has a client census of 12–15.

On one particularly busy day shift, Katie, who is working short-staffed, gives the wrong medications to a post-hysterectomy client. She completes an incident report form, calls the attending physician, and monitors the client closely for any unusual effects. The following day, the client is discharged home without any obvious complications from the medication error.

One month later, Katie receives a notice that she is being called in for a deposition related to a malpractice suit naming her as a codefendant with the hospital. The client who was given the wrong medications has claimed partial paralysis as a result of the error.

Even though Katie did in fact commit a medication error, the client must prove a cause-and-effect relationship between the error and the injury. In order to do this, all potential causes must be considered. For example, is there a likelihood that paralysis could occur as a side effect of the medications? Has the client experienced a change in her condition that could explain the paralysis? In other words, the plaintiff must prove that Katie's error of commission is the direct cause of the injury.

One of the most common malpractice charges of omission is that of failing to report a client's changing condition to the appropriate physician. Nurses are expected to ensure that clients receive safe and competent care. If a client's health status worsens and a nurse fails to seek medical attention, that nurse has breached a duty to the client (Bernzweig, 1996). On the other hand, a nurse who does not challenge an inappropriate physician order may also be considered negligent.

Confidentiality

Clients have a right to expect nurses to safeguard personal information shared as part of the nurse–client relationship; that is, they have a right to confidentiality. This means client information should not be discussed without the client's consent in elevators, the hospital cafeteria, and in conversations with friends away from work. Treatment records should not be released to a third party without the client's written consent. Information should be shared only with those members of the health care team who are involved in planning and delivering care to the client.

Nurses are prohibited from divulging client information by institutional policies and state and federal laws, and are expected to follow ethical principles described in the American Nurses' Association Code of Ethics. Clients should be able to rely on nurses to protect their personal affairs from unwanted scrutiny by others. Failure to protect a client's confidential information carries potential ethical and legal ramifications for a nurse.

Exceptions to client confidentiality do exist in some situations, however. Most states have passed laws that require the mandatory disclosure (or duty to report) of such occurrences as gunshot wounds, child abuse, attempted suicide, and threats to third parties (Betts, 2001).

Informed Consent

In a landmark Supreme Court case, *Schloendorff v. Society of New York Hospitals* (1914), Justice Benjamin Cardozo held that "every human being of adult years and sound mind has a right to determine what will be done with his own body" (p. 93). Since that time, laws have firmly established what information should be shared with clients in order for them to make the best possible decisions regarding their health care.

Nurses, because of the nature of their work, are often called upon to witness clients' signatures on permission forms for procedures. The physician is responsible for explaining all procedures and expected outcomes to the client. It is especially important that clients receive and understand all necessary information prior to agreeing to the procedure, such as risks, benefits, potential complications, cost, and alternatives (Betts, 2001). Equally important are the following conditions of **informed consent**:

- Consent must be given voluntarily by the client or his/her designee.
- The person giving consent must have the mental capacity to understand (competence).

If at all possible, the client should be the one to give informed consent. When clients are minors, are mentally incapable, or have other limitations that inhibit their full capacity to comprehend instructions and make a decision, the next of kin or a court-appointed proxy may give consent.

The nurse is responsible for determining that the client fully understands the information, and should strive to support his/her decision regarding consent. A client should never be pressured to sign a consent form if he or she has reservations. The physician should be contacted to clarify any of the client's questions or concerns.

Assault and Battery

If health care procedures or activities are performed without the client's consent, the intentional tort of assault and/or battery has occurred. **Assault** is a threat

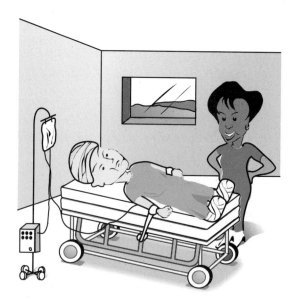

Figure 10-1
Use care in restraining clients.

or attempt to make bodily contact with another person without permission. **Battery** is the actual unpermitted touching of one person by another (Betts, 2001). Actual harm does not have to occur for a claim to be filed against a nurse for assault and battery.

On occasion, a nurse may consider forced care to be in the best interest of the client. Sometimes, for example, a client who refuses to get out of bed may be lifted out of the bed and placed in a bedside chair. This simple act constitutes battery if the client does not agree to the physical contact.

It is imperative that nurses remember that clients have the right to refuse care, even if it is "in their best interests." A client should never be threatened with unauthorized contact (Figure 10–1). How often do nurses tell clients they will be restrained if they do not remain in bed? Such restraint is, in fact and in law, **false imprisonment.** Unfortunately, many nurses tend to use their relationship with clients as a means to dictate care, rather than work in cooperation with clients and families.

RISK MANAGEMENT

The process of identifying, evaluating, and reducing actual or potential legal problems in a health care setting is called **risk management** (Brent, 1998). Nurses can take steps to prevent many liability claims by following these suggestions:

1. Familiarize yourself with your agency's policies and procedures. If you are unsure about the steps of a procedure, look it up before proceeding any further. By practicing in a manner inconsistent with established protocols, you expose yourself to needless liability.
2. Listen to what your clients are telling you, and take immediate actions to meet their needs. Evaluate clients carefully for changes in condition, and notify the appropriate health care professional for assistance in providing care. Follow up with the client after interventions to relieve pain, prevent falls, and so forth.
3. If you have difficulty obtaining physician help to care for a client whose condition is worsening, notify the appropriate supervisor and follow all chains of command until the client receives the needed help. Continue to closely monitor and provide necessary interventions for the client, and document carefully all findings, care, and phone calls on the client's behalf.
4. Do not take shortcuts in charting. Good documentation is the nurse's best ally in a lawsuit. By taking time to chart appropriate assessments, interventions, and evaluations of care, you will provide yourself with a careful accounting of client care activities in case of litigation.
5. Take precautions to ensure client safety. Keep side rails up and beds in low positions when indicated. Have spills on floors cleaned up immediately, and encourage clients to wear nonslip shoes when out of bed. Make sure

all equipment is kept in good repair. Assist clients during transfers from beds to wheelchairs, stretchers, and when ambulating.

6. Remain especially alert during medication administration. Avoid distractions such as questions from others while preparing medications. Be sure to observe the Five Rights of medications administration: (1) right medication, (2) right dose, (3) right route, (4) right client, (5) right time. Pay particular attention when giving medications that carry a higher rate of error during administration, such as heparin, insulin, potassium, and chemotherapy (Fiesta, 1998).

7. Listen to your clients. They may question a medication that looks unfamiliar, or may be trying to tell you about a significant problem. They may not understand the correct medical terminology to use, but can provide you with important cues to prevent errors.

8. Practice a healthy lifestyle that will help you to feel your best while at work. If you are distracted by fatigue, illness, or personal worries, you are much more likely to make errors.

9. Carry personal liability insurance. If you are sued and have malpractice insurance, you will be more likely to have your own attorney (and thus more control over your own welfare) than if not. Hospitals and other health care agencies usually have insurance to cover nurses in the event of a lawsuit; however, they would retain the control over a decision about settling out of court or going before a jury. You, as the employee of the agency, would have little input without your own insurance.

Nurses typically participate in the employing agency's risk management activities by providing information regarding difficulties experienced during client care (Brent, 1998). One way to communicate such information is by documenting unusual happenings so action may be taken to avoid future occurrences. Sometimes referred to as an **incident report,** the information serves as an actual accounting of the details of the event. These reports are widely used for quality improvement activities and are typically kept separate from the client's chart.

Nursing is undeniably a profession where a multitude of legal concerns exist. By practicing safe, proactive client care, the nurse will be in a better position to avoid litigation.

VALUES AND ETHICS IN NURSING

Nurses strive to meet human needs; but because of the nature of the decisions they must make daily, they can have either a positive or negative impact on client care outcomes. Clients, families, and communities have expectations of receiving nursing care that is competent, compassionate, and supportive. For nurses to meet these expectations, they must first understand their own value systems and they must be familiar with the basic ethical theories and principles used to guide practice.

Values

Values are beliefs and attitudes about what is important to a person. For example, you may value honesty and a strong work ethic. Someone else might stress fairness and loyalty. We tend to choose those things that are of significance to us based on the influence of others in our lives. If, for example, your parents emphasized civic responsibility as a desirable trait, it's more than likely that you will too.

The ANA Code of Ethics (Box 10–2) outlines desirable ethical behaviors for nurses, such as safeguarding clients' rights to privacy and protecting the public from unethical practice. Jean Watson (1979), a leading nursing theorist

---

Box 10-2   *American Nurses Association Code of Ethics*

---

1. The nurse provides services with respect for human dignity and the uniqueness of the client unrestricted by considerations of social or economic status, personal attributes, or the nature of health problems.
2. The nurse safeguards the client's right to privacy by judiciously protecting information of a confidential nature.
3. The nurse acts to safeguard the client and the public when health care and safety are affected by the incompetent, unethical, or illegal practice of any person.
4. The nurse assumes responsibility and accountability for individual nursing judgments and actions.
5. The nurse maintains competence in nursing.
6. The nurse exercises informed judgment and uses individual competence and qualifications as criteria in seeking consultation, accepting responsibilities, and delegating nursing activities to others.
7. The nurse participates in activities that contribute to the ongoing development of the profession's body of knowledge.
8. The nurse participates in the profession's efforts to implement and improve standards of nursing.
9. The nurse participates in the profession's efforts to establish and maintain conditions of employment conducive to high-quality nursing care.
10. The nurse participates in the profession's efforts to protect the public from misinformation and misrepresentation and to maintain the integrity of nursing.
11. The nurse collaborates with members of the health professions and other citizens in promoting community and national efforts to meet the health needs of the public.

Reprinted with permission from *Code for nurses with interpretive statements.* © 1985. Washington DC: American Nurses Publishing, American Nurses Foundation/American Nurses Association.

on nursing and caring, supports this Code by suggesting that members of the nursing profession should possess the following values:

- a strong commitment to service
- belief in the dignity and worth of each person
- a commitment to continuing education
- autonomy

As you are probably aware, clients do not always share your value system. For example, let's say you are pro-life. Suppose an 18-year-old unmarried woman comes into your agency seeking an abortion. Answer the following questions:

How would your beliefs about abortion influence your nurse–client relationship?

_____

_____

_____

_____

_____

_____

Could you put your feelings aside and respect her right to choose? If so, describe how.

_____

_____

_____

_____

_____

_____

Clarification of your personal values is the first step in preparing to care for clients who are experiencing ethically challenging situations. Nurses should strive to set aside judgmental feelings and personal beliefs in order to support each client to make the best decisions. As you gain experience and develop more competence as a nurse, you may find that your own values change, and that you will actually become more tolerant of the beliefs and lifestyles of others.

Ethical Principles

A set of principles is used to determine moral obligations, or what is correct and incorrect in particular situations. The following ethical principles are common to client care: (1) autonomy, (2) veracity, (3) beneficence, (4) nonmaleficence, (5) justice, and (6) fidelity.

Autonomy refers to a client's right to make his or her own decision without coercion. Nurses should respect the client's autonomy and remember that clients may not always make choices in their own best interests. For example, an adult client may refuse to have a blood transfusion because of religious beliefs, despite a slim chance of survival without it. The client's decision should always be honored, regardless of a nurse's personal beliefs about this issue.

Veracity is the duty to tell the truth, and may become an issue for nurses when clients ask questions about their diagnoses, treatments, and so forth. Nurses are obligated to be truthful; and, as a rule, the client should be given as much information as possible regarding care (Katims, 1998). Occasionally, family members ask nurses to withhold negative medical information from clients, presumably because it could be upsetting. The client has the right to expect to be kept completely informed about his or her medical condition.

Beneficence, or "doing good" involves caring for clients in a manner that will promote their welfare, whereas nonmaleficence refers to avoiding harm to clients, whether intentional or unintentional. These two ethical principles tend to overlap in actual practice, since nurses typically attempt to uphold both simultaneously.

The principle justice refers to treating all people fairly. For example, clients should not be discriminated against because of cultural beliefs incongruent with those of health care providers. All clients have the right to expect the same level of care. In addition, a critically ill client should not be denied health care because of an inability to pay.

Finally, fidelity is the duty to be faithful to commitments. If you tell a client you will not divulge confidential information to his family members, then you must keep that promise. Can you see a similarity between the ethical term fidelity and the legal term confidentiality? The violation of ethical principles may involve the nurse in eventual litigation in some instances (Figure 10–2).

Ethical Theories

Two main theoretical stances that dominate discussions surrounding ethical issues in nursing are *deontology* and *teleology*. These theories establish defined guidelines, or norms, upon which to base decisions.

Deontology is based on the premise that all life is worthy of respect. This theory assumes that all humans have the "freedom, thoughtfulness, and sensibility to act in a moral manner" (Katims, 1998, p. 46). In other words, right or wrong is clearly based on one's duty or obligation to follow moral rules. Deontol-

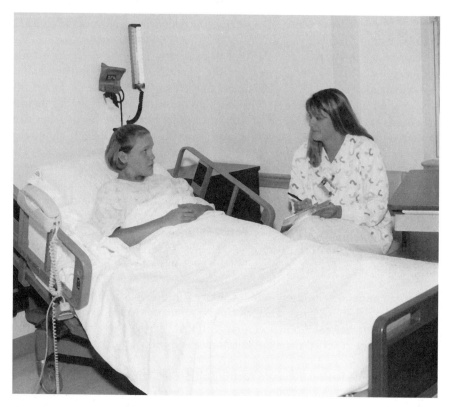

Figure 10-2
Nurses have a duty to keep client information confidential.

ogy supports veracity, client autonomy, and justice. The following scenario utilizes deontological thinking:

> Meredith is a client who has cancer of the esophagus. She has taken a maximum dose of narcotics for pain and is calling the nurse's station for more medication. The unit charge nurse goes to Meredith's room to speak with her. She finds Meredith crying and requesting to be given an overdose of medication to end her pain. Meredith says she would "just like to die right now and get it over with." The nurse explains to Meredith that she will do all she can to help make her comfortable, but cannot assist with suicide for personal ethical and legal reasons.

Teleology is an approach to ethical decisions based on the following premise: That which is useful is good. In other words, an emphasis is placed on results, not moral principles of right and wrong. The greatest happiness for the greatest number of people is more important than individual happiness. Consider this scenario, which uses a teleological form of reasoning:

> Jordan is a ten-year-old who is awaiting a liver transplant. He has been in ICU for several days, and his parents have been told that their health insurance policy has been canceled because Jordan has reached the maximum allowed coverage. A member of the transplant health care team visits with Jordan's parents the next day to make plans to discharge him home, since hospital care will no longer be paid for by insurance. His parents are informed that Jordan will receive continuing care at home under the direction of home care nurses in order to keep his health care costs down and to provide an ICU bed for more acute clients.

Since ethical problems are complex, many nurses feel that neither theory can be applied exclusively to everyday clinical practice. A common practice is to use a situational approach to ethical problem solving (Katims, 1998; Pappas, 1997). This view allows for each situation to create its own set of rules depending on the circumstances. For example, euthanasia may seem acceptable for a 92-year-old ventilator-dependent woman who is a quadriplegic, but not a 30-year-old woman with breast cancer.

A recent theme in nursing literature has been that of an ethics of care. The works of Nel Noddings (1984), Carol Gilligan (1982), and nursing theorist Jean Watson (1979) have emphasized the caring aspect of the nurse–client relationship as the cornerstone for ethical decision making. In order to determine what is best for the client, the nurse enters into a caring, compassionate relationship with the client, who develops trust and confidence in the nurse as a caregiver.

ETHICAL DILEMMAS AND DECISION MAKING

Ethical principles and theories provide the groundwork for ethical decision making with clients; however, they do not provide clearcut answers for difficult situations. An **ethical dilemma** arises when a choice must be made between conflicting values, issues, or principles, and both choices are equally unsatisfactory (Pappas, 1997). The following is an example of an ethical dilemma.

> A 43-year-old male client has been admitted for stomach pain and learns that he has AIDS. He asks the nurse to keep the diagnosis from his wife and children. As the client is being prepared for discharge, his wife approaches the nurse outside the client's hearing and asks if something is wrong that she has not been told.

What do you think the nurse should do? Why? What ethical principles are in conflict, if any?

_____

_____

_____

_____

_____

Are there legal as well as ethical considerations here? What are they?

_____

_____

_____

_____

_____

Such problems have no easy solutions; however, the use of an ethical decision making framework can greatly assist the nurse. Figure 10–3 shows a step-by-step process for ethical decision making. Recognition of a problem of an ethical

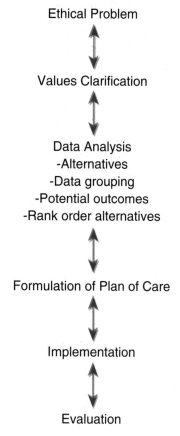

Figure 10-3
Ethical decision making framework.

nature is the first step in the process, and involves obtaining a clear picture of what is occurring. The problem must be specifically stated, without speculation or conjecture as to what might be happening.

Next, all aspects of the problem must be clearly identified. All sources and participants involved in the situation must be tapped for thorough data collection. It is imperative that nurses use good observation, assessment, and recording skills.

Before proceeding further, nurses must be willing to analyze personal values to prevent bias during participation in ethical decision making with clients. There should be no conflict of interest on the part of the nurse, and she should be able to avoid being influenced by preconceived notions. Nurses should be able to focus solely on the client's best interests and resist the urge to give advice based on personal feelings.

Analysis of data consists of four steps: (1) identifying various alternatives, (2) grouping of data, (3) formulating potential client outcomes, and (4) rank ordering of alternatives. The identification of possible alternatives should include all feasible choices available to the client. Information gathered from the client, family, and others is grouped under the alternative to which it best corresponds. From these clusters, formulation of potential client outcomes for each alternative may occur. The last step in data analysis is the rank ordering of alternatives on a scale from the most to least beneficial to the client.

Following data analysis, the client and family should work with the nurse to develop a plan of care based on the alternative that has the most merit. Care must be taken to carefully choose the best course of action with the fewest number of negative consequences.

Once the plan of care has been implemented, the final step in the framework is one of evaluation. This is perhaps one of the most important components of the process, and involves evaluation of the outcomes and revision of the plan as needed.

You may be wondering if nurses actually have the time to use a framework of this sort in practice. At first glance, it appears lengthy and confusing; on closer scrutiny, however, it is similar to the steps of the nursing process (see chapter 7), which is familiar to nurses.

Now let's apply the framework to an ethical dilemma:

> Lela Martin is a 92-year-old female who has chronic obstructive lung disease. She has had numerous hospitalizations for respiratory failure, each of which resulted in her being placed on a ventilator for several weeks. Lela recently talked with her private physician and made the decision to refuse any resuscitative measures in the future. She completed the necessary paperwork with her attorney and submitted signed copies to her physician and the local hospital.
>
> Early one Saturday morning, Lela became very dyspneic and anxious. She summoned her neighbor for help, who immediately called an ambulance to take Lela to the hospital. During the trip, Lela became unconscious.

Hospital staff called Lela's daughter to the Emergency Department when they discovered her signed form indicating her preference to refuse any lifesaving measures. Martha Lincoln, Lela's daughter, became very angry and demanded that the Emergency Department staff "do everything possible to save her or I will sue you!"

Consider yourself the Emergency Department nurse in this situation. By using the ethical decision making framework in Figure 10–3, we can outline the process as follows:

Ethical Problem

An ethical dilemma exists because the ethical principles of autonomy (client's wishes for self-determination) and beneficence ("do good" for the daughter, help her preserve her mother's life) are in conflict. As a nurse, you want to honor the wishes of both the client and her daughter.

Values Clarification

Upon analysis of your personal value system, you determine that you believe in the sanctity of life, but do not want to see the client suffer needlessly due to futile efforts to prolong her life. You also believe clients have the right to self-determination.

Data Analysis

Alternative 1

Honor the client's wishes

Data:

- the client has an advance directive document to support her wishes
- the client has past experiences with resuscitation, so has knowledge of the consequences

Potential Outcomes:

- you preserve the client's right to autonomy
- you risk a lawsuit from the client's daughter

Alternative 2

Honor the daughter's wishes

Data:

- the daughter was not aware of her mother's request for no resuscitative measures
- the daughter expresses a desire to discuss the content of the advance directive with her mother, so wants her oxygenated and conscious
- the daughter believes her mother should have every chance to be cured of this disease

Potential Outcomes:

- the daughter will have a chance to speak with her mother and clarify her mother's wishes
- the client will be angry and could seek legal action

Rank Ordering of Alternatives

1. Honor the client's wishes
2. Honor the daughter's wishes

Rationale for Rank Ordering

The nurse and physician choose to honor the client's wishes since the advance directive clearly state the desire for no resuscitation. At the time of the client's decision, she consciously sought help from an attorney and informed both the private physician and hospital of her choice. Even though the daughter may seek legal action against the nurse, other members of the health care team, and the hospital, the client's wishes are the most important.

Formulation of Plan of Care

The nurse plans to go with the physician to speak with the daughter in a private area. They will inform the daughter of the decision to honor the client's request on the advance directive.

Implementation of Plan of Care

The nurse and health care team use all possible comfort care measures for both the client and her daughter to assist them through this acute episode. The daughter will require an explanation as to why the client's decision was upheld, and should be treated in a caring, understanding manner. Other professionals may be called upon to assist the daughter during this time, such as the family minister, other family members, and friends. If the client regains consciousness and is able to talk with her daughter, allow uninterrupted time for them to be alone.

Evaluation

Monitor the outcomes of the plan by analyzing the daughter's response to the decision and the client's response to comfort care measures. If the daughter continues to be angry, support from a member of hospital administration may be needed.

Ethical dilemmas are a challenging aspect of nursing practice, and can cause much uncertainty and confusion in the mind of even the most experienced nurse. Despite a basic understanding of ethical theories and principles, nurses continue to report feelings of powerlessness in such situations (Pappas, 1997). The use of a framework for ethical decision making may be a helpful tool to assist nurses in organizing data and formulating solutions.

CURRENT BIOETHICAL ISSUES

From the preceding case, it may seem as if ethical decision making involves primarily health care professionals, the client, and the family. In actuality, ethical decisions are influenced by various societal and legal factors. Many changes are occurring in today's world, and nurses are constantly challenged by new problems. Individual rights have become more important in all aspects of living and dying. The focus of health care has shifted from a disease-based system to one of health promotion and disease prevention.

Because of technological advances and changing attitudes toward individual rights, nurses are being called upon to care for clients who are faced with bioethical issues that were undreamed of but a few decades ago. Two major categories encompass the majority of today's bioethical concerns: (1) issues created by new technology and (2) concerns raised by a client's right to self-determination.

Scientific breakthroughs have allowed for the creation and prolongation of life by artificial means. Artificial insemination and surrogate motherhood have presented childless couples with the opportunity to become parents. While a blessing in some ways, new reproductive procedures have raised difficult legal/ ethical questions. Who, for example, has the legal right to be called a surrogate child's *mother*—the egg donor or the woman who carries and gives birth to the child? What should be done with fertilized eggs not used during *in vitro* fertilization?

While advances in transplant surgery have saved lives, ethical concerns surrounding equity in care have been raised. Who decides which client should receive organs that are in short supply? Should a client with health insurance be chosen over one who cannot pay for the surgery?

Another issue is that of *futile care*—the use of medical interventions without hope of benefit to the client (Pappas, 1997). The focus of the medical profession has long been to preserve life; sometimes, however, client's lives are being lengthened when there is very little chance for improvement. Always an emotional issue, the debate over whether or not to use every possible means to save a life involves health care team members, clients, their families, and a society faced with bearing the cost.

Because of a number of widely publicized cases of dispute between families and health care providers over the use of life support, the **Patient Self-Determination Act** was passed in 1991. This act mandates that health care agencies inform clients of their right to choose which life-prolonging treatment options they desire in the event that they should later be incapable of making a decision. Legal, written instructions known as **advance directives** become a part of a client's legal record.

Bioethical issues pertaining to the client's right to self-determination include euthanasia, physician-assisted suicide, and abortion. Many unanswered questions remain in regard to whether a person has the legal/ethical right to choose when to end his/her life or when and how to terminate a pregnancy.

As you pursue your career in nursing, legal/ethical issues will continue to change as societal attitudes and pressures influence health care. Many nurses experience frustration and uncertainty when confronted with client problems of this sort. Even though many situations have no easy answer, always try to choose a course of action that is in the best interest of the client.

As you assume more responsibility for client management, it is essential that you understand legal/ethical considerations associated with nursing practice. Remember to seek support from other peers, supervisors, agency ethics committees, and legal advisors. You are not solely responsible for helping clients make difficult ethical decisions; however, you will be ultimately held accountable for your actions.

CRITICAL THINKING EXERCISES

1. Examine your state's nurse practice act and describe how you believe it will influence your personal practice as a registered nurse.

   _____

   _____

   _____

   _____

   _____

   _____

2. If possible, describe a client care situation from personal experience in which you believe assault and/or battery occurred. How could this have been prevented? How will you approach this type of situation in the future?

_____

_____

_____

_____

_____

_____

3. Develop a plan of care for a belligerent client who is sedated and refuses to stay in bed, taking into account risk management considerations.

_____

_____

_____

_____

_____

_____

4. Describe an ethically difficult situation that you have encountered in practice. Identify at least two ethical principles that were in conflict and discuss how this dilemma was resolved.

_____

_____

_____

_____

_____

_____

5. Apply the ethical decision making framework from Figure 10–3 to the situation in question 4. Is your solution different from what actually occurred? How?

_____

_____

_____

_____

_____

_____

REFERENCES

Bernzeig, E. (1996). *The nurse's liability for malpractice* (6th ed.). St. Louis: C.V. Mosby.

Betts, V. (2001). Legal aspects of nursing. In *Professional nursing: Concepts and challenges* (3rd ed.), K. Chitty, ed. Philadelphia: W.B. Saunders.

Brent, N. (1998). Legal implications in nursing. In *Foundations of nursing practice: A nursing process approach*, J. Leahy and P. Kizilay, eds. Philadelphia: W.B. Saunders.

Fiesta, J. (1998). Legal aspects of medication administration. *Nursing Management* 29(1):22–23.

Gilligan, C. (1982). *In a different voice: Psychological theory and women's development.* Cambridge: Harvard University Press.

Hall, J. (1996). *Nursing ethics and law.* Philadelphia: W.B. Saunders.

Katims, I. (1998). Values and ethics in nursing practice. In *Foundations of nursing practice: A nursing process approach*, J. Leahy and P. Kizilay, eds. Philadelphia: W.B. Saunders.

Noddings, N. (1984). *Caring: A feminine approach to ethics and moral education.* Berkeley: University of California Press.

Pappas, A. (1997). Ethical issues. In *Nursing today: Transition and trends* (2nd ed.), J. Zerwekh and J. Claborn, eds. Philadelphia: W.B. Saunders.

Schloendorff v. Society of New York Hospitals, 105 N.E. 92 (1914).

Sheehan, J. (1997). Safeguard your license: The disciplinary process. *RN* 60(1):53–55, 58–59.

Stark, S. (1997). Legal issues. In *Nursing today: Transition and trends* (2nd ed.), J. Zerwekh and J. Claborn, eds. Philadelphia: W.B. Saunders.

Watson, J. (1979). *Nursing—The philosophy and science of caring.* Boston: Little, Brown.

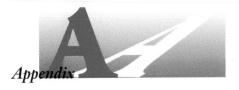

State Boards of Nursing

NOTE: These addresses and Websites were current as of May 2001.

Alabama
Alabama Board of Nursing
RSA Plaza, Suite 250
770 Washington Avenue
P.O. Box 303900
Montgomery, Alabama 36130-3900
Phone: (334) 242-4060
Fax: (334) 242-4360
http://www.abn.state.al.us/

Alaska
Alaska Board of Nursing
Department of Community and
    Economic Development
Division of Occupational Licensing
3601 C Street, Suite 722
Anchorage, Alaska 99503
Phone: (907) 269-8161
Fax: (907) 269-8196
http://www.dced.state.ak.us/occ/
    pnur.htm
Mailing address:
P.O. Box 110806
Juneau, Alaska 99811-0806

American Samoa
American Samoa Health Services
    Regulatory Board
LBJ Tropical Medical Center
Pago Pago, American Samoa 96799

Phone: 011-(684) 633-1222
Fax: 011-(684) 633-1869

Arizona
Arizona State Board of Nursing
1651 E. Morten Avenue, Suite 150
Phoenix, Arizona 85020
Phone: (602) 331-8111
Fax: (602) 906-9365
http://azboardofnursing.org/

Arkansas
Arkansas State Board of Nursing
University Tower Building, Suite 800
1123 South University
Little Rock, Arkansas 72204
Phone: (501) 686-2700
Fax: (501) 686-2714
http://www.state.ar.us/nurse

California—RN
California Board of Registered
    Nursing
400 R Street, Suite 4030
Sacramento, California 95814-6239
Phone: (916) 322-3350
Fax: (916) 327-4402
http://www.rn.ca.gov/

Colorado
Colorado Board of Nursing
1560 Broadway, Suite 880

Denver, Colorado 80202
Phone: (303) 894-2430
Fax: (303) 894-2821

http://www.dora.state.co.us/nursing/

Connecticut
Connecticut Board of Examiners for
    Nursing
Division of Health Systems
    Regulation
410 Capital Avenue, MS # 13PHO
P.O. Box 340308
Hartford, Connecticut 06134-0328
Phone: (860) 509-7624
Fax: (860) 509-7553

http://www.state.ct.us/dph/

Delaware
Delaware Board of Nursing
861 Silver Lake Boulevard
Cannon Building, Suite 203
Dover, Delaware 19904
Phone: (302) 739-4522
Fax: (302) 739-2711

District of Columbia
District of Columbia Board of
    Nursing
Department of Health
825 N. Capitol Street, N.E.
    2nd floor, Room 2224
Washington, DC 20002
Phone: (202) 442-4778
Fax: (202) 442-9431

Florida
Florida Board of Nursing
4080 Woodcock Drive, Suite 202
Jacksonville, Florida 32207
Phone: (904) 858-6940
Fax: (904) 858-6964

http://www.myflorida.com/mqa/

Georgia—RN
Georgia Board of Nursing
237 Coliseum Drive
Macon, Georgia 31217-3858
Phone: (912) 207-1640
Fax: (912) 207-1660

http://www.sos.state.ga.us/ebd-rn/

Guam
Guam Board of Nurse Examiners
P.O. Box 2816
1304 East Sunset Boulevard
Barrgada, Guam 96913
Phone: 011-(671) 475-0251
Fax: 011-(671) 477-4733

Hawaii
Hawaii Board of Nursing
Professional and Vocational
    Licensing Division
P.O. Box 3469
Honolulu, Hawaii 96801
Phone: (808) 586-3000
Fax: (808) 586-2689

Idaho
Idaho Board of Nursing
280 N. 8th Street,
    Suite 210
P.O. Box 83720
Boise, Idaho 83720
Phone: (208) 334-3110
Fax: (208) 334-3262

http://www.state.id.us/ibn/
    ibnhome.htm

Illinois
Illinois Department of Professional
    Regulation
James R. Thompson Center
100 West Randolph, Suite 9-300
Chicago, Illinois 60601

Phone: (312) 814-2715
Fax: (312) 814-3145
http://www.dpr.state.il.us/

Indiana
Indiana State Board of Nursing
Health Professions Bureau
402 West Washington Street
Room W041
Indianapolis, Indiana 46204
Phone: (317) 232-2960
Fax: (317) 233-4236

http://www.ai.org/hpb

Iowa
Iowa Board of Nursing
RiverPoint Business Park
400 SW 8th Street, Suite B
Des Moines, Iowa 50309-4685
Phone: (515) 281-3255
Fax: (515) 281-4825

http://www.state.ia.us/government/
    nursing/

Kansas
Kansas State Board of Nursing
Landon State Office Building
900 S.W. Jackson, Suite 551-S
Topeka, Kansas 66612-1230
Phone: (785) 296-4929
Fax: (785) 296-3929

http://www.ksbn.org/

Kentucky
Kentucky Board of Nursing
312 Whittington Parkway, Suite 300
Louisville, Kentucky 40222
Phone: (502) 329-7000
Fax: (502) 329-7011

http://www.kbn.state.ky.us/

Louisiana—RN
Louisiana State Board of Nursing
3510 N. Causeway Boulevard,
    Suite 501

Metairie, Louisiana 70003
Phone: (504) 838-5332
Fax: (504) 838-5349

http://www/lsbn.state.la.us/

Maine
Maine State Board of Nursing
158 State House Station
Augusta, Maine 04333
Phone: (207) 287-1133
Fax: (207) 287-1149

http://www.state.me.us/nursingbd/

Maryland
Maryland Board of Nursing
4140 Patterson Avenue
Baltimore, Maryland 21215
Phone: (410) 585-1900
Fax: (410) 358-3530

http://dhmh.state.md.us/mbn/

Massachusetts
Massachusetts Board of Registration
    in Nursing
Commonwealth of Massachusetts
239 Causeway Street
Boston, MA 02114
Phone: (617) 727-9961
Fax: (617) 727-1630

http://www.state.ma.us/reg/
    boards/rn/default.htm

Michigan
Michigan CIS/Office of Health
    Services
Ottawa Towers North
611 West Ottawa, 4th floor
Lansing, Michigan 48933
Phone: (517) 373-9102
Fax: (517) 373-2179

http://www.cis.state.mi.us/bhser/
    genover.htm

Minnesota
Minnesota Board of Nursing
2829 University Avenue SE, Suite 500
Minneapolis, Minnesota 55414
Phone: (612) 617-2270
Fax: (612) 617-2190
http://www.nursingboard.state.mn.us/

Mississippi
Mississippi Board of Nursing
1935 Lakeland Drive, Suite B
Jackson, Mississippi 39216
Phone: (601) 987-4188
Fax: (601) 364-2352

Missouri
Missouri State Board of Nursing
3605 Missouri Boulevard
P.O. Box 656
Jefferson City, Missouri 65102-0656
Phone: (573) 751-0681
Fax: (573) 751-0075
http://www.ecodev.state.mo.us/pr/nursing/

Montana
Montana State Board of Nursing
301 South Park
Helena, Montana 59620-0513
Phone: (406) 444-2071
Fax: (406) 871-2343
http://www.com.state.mt.us/license/pol/pol__boards/nur__board/board__page.htm

Nebraska
Nebraska Health and Human Services System
Department of Regulation and Licensure, Nursing Section
301 Centennial Mall South

P.O. Box 94986
Lincoln, Nebraska 68509-4986
Phone: (402) 471-4376
Fax: (402) 471-3577
http://www.hhs.state.ne.us/crl/nns.htm

Nevada
Nevada State Board of Nursing (Las Vegas area)
4330 S. Valley View, Suite 106
Las Vegas, Nevada 89103
Phone: (702) 486-5800
Fax: (702) 486-5803

Nevada State Board of Nursing (Reno/Carson City area)
1755 East Plumb Lane, Suite 260
Reno, Nevada 89502
Phone: (775) 688-2620
Fax: (775) 688-2628
http://www.nursingboard.state.nv.us/

New Hampshire
New Hampshire Board of Nursing
78 Regional Drive, BLDG B
P.O. Box 3898
Concord, New Hampshire 03302
Phone: (603) 271-2323
Fax: (603) 271-6605
http://www.state.nh.us/nursing/

New Jersey
New Jersey Board of Nursing
124 Halsey Street, 6th floor
P.O. Box 45010
Newark, New Jersey 07101
Phone: (973) 504-6586
Fax: (973) 648-3481
http://www.state.nj.us/lps/ca/medical.htm

New Mexico
New Mexico Board of Nursing
4206 Louisiana Boulevard, NE,
    Suite A
Albuquerque, New Mexico 87109
Phone: (505) 841-8340
Fax: (505) 841-8347

http://www.state.nm.us/clients/
    nursing

New York
New York State Board of Nursing
Education Building
89 Washington Avenue, 2nd floor,
    West Wing
Albany, New York 12234
Phone: (518) 473-6999
Fax: (518) 474-3706

http://www.nysed.gov/prof/
    nurse.htm

North Carolina
North Carolina Board of Nursing
3724 National Drive, Suite 201
P.O. Box 2129
Raleigh, North Carolina 27612
Phone: (919) 782-3211
Fax: (919) 781-9461

http://www.ncbon.com/

North Dakota
North Dakota Board of Nursing
919 South 7th Street, Suite 504
Bismarck, North Dakota 58504
Phone: (701) 328-9777
Fax: (701) 328-9785

http://www.ndbon.org/

Northern Mariana Islands
Commonwealth Board of Nurse
    Examiners
Public Health Center
P.O. Box 1458

Saipan, MP 96950
Phone: 011-(670) 234-8950
Fax: 011-(670) 234-8930

Ohio
Ohio Board of Nursing
17 South High Street, Suite 400
Columbus, Ohio 43215-3413
Phone: (614) 466-3947
Fax: (614) 466-0388

http://www.state.oh.us/nur/

Oklahoma
Oklahoma Board of Nursing
2915 North Classen Boulevard,
    Suite 524
Oklahoma City, Oklahoma 73106
Phone: (405) 962-1800
Fax: (405) 962-1821

Oregon
Oregon State Board of Nursing
Suite 465
800 NE Oregon Street, Box 25
Portland, Oregon 97232
Phone: (503) 731-4745
Fax: (503) 731-4755

http://www.osbn.state.or.us/

Pennsylvania
Pennsylvania State Board of Nursing
124 Pine Street
P.O. Box 2649
Harrisburg, Pennsylvania 17101
Phone: (717) 783-7142
Fax: (717) 787-0822

http://www.dos.state.pa.us/bpoa/
    nurbd/mainpage.htm

Puerto Rico
Commonwealth of Puerto Rico
    Board of Nurse Examiners
800 Roberto H. Todd Avenue

Room 202, Stop 18
Santurce, Puerto Rico 00908
Phone: (787) 725-8161
Fax: (787) 725-7903

Rhode Island
Rhode Island Board of Nurse
    Registration & Nursing
    Education
105 Cannon Building
Three Capitol Hill
Providence, Rhode Island 02908-
    5097
Phone: (401) 222-5700
Fax: (401) 222-3352

South Carolina
South Carolina State Board of
    Nursing
110 Centerview Drive, Suite 202
Columbia, South Carolina 29210
Phone: (803) 896-4550
Fax: (803) 896-4525

http://www.llr.state.sc.us/POL/
    nursing/default.htm
Mailing address:
P.O. Box 12367
Columbia, SC 29211

South Dakota
South Dakota Board of Nursing
4300 South Louise Avenue,
    Suite C-1
Sioux Falls, South Dakota 57106-
    3124
Phone: (605) 362-2760
Fax: (605) 362-2768

http://www.state.sd.us/dcr/nursing/

Tennessee
Tennessee State Board of Nursing
426 Fifth Avenue North

1st floor—Cordell Hull Building
Nashville, Tennessee 37247
Phone: (615) 532-5166
Fax: (615) 741-7899

http://170.142.76.180/bmf-bin/
    BMFproflist.pl

Texas—RN
Texas Board of Nurse Examiners
William P. Hobby Building,
    Tower 3
333 Guadalupe, Suite 3-460
Austin, Texas 78701
Phone: (512) 305-7400
Fax: (512) 305-7401

http://www.bne.state.tx.us/
Mailing Address:
P.O. Box 430
Austin, Texas 78716-0430

Utah
Utah State Board of Nursing
Heber M. Wells Building,
    4th floor
160 East 300 South
Salt Lake City, Utah 84111
Phone: (801) 530-6628
Fax: (801) 530-6511

http://www.commerce.state.ut.us/

Vermont
Vermont State Board of Nursing
109 State Street
Montpelier, Vermont 05609-1106
Phone: (802) 828-2396
Fax: (802) 828-2484

http://vtprofessionals.org/nurses/
Mailing Address:
26 Terrace Street
Drawer 9
Montpelier, Vermont 05609-1101

Virgin Islands
Virgin Islands Board of Nurse
   Licensure
Veterans Drive Station
St. Thomas, U.S. Virgin Islands
   00803
Phone: (340) 776-7397
Fax: (340) 777-4003

Virginia
Virginia Board of Nursing
6606 West Broad Street, 4th floor
Richmond, Virginia 23230
Phone: (804) 662-9909
Fax: (804) 662-9512

http://www.dhp.state.va.us/nursing/

Washington
Washington State Nursing Care
   Quality Assurance Commission
Department of Health
1300 Quince Street SE
Olympia, Washington 98504-7864
Phone: (360) 236-4740
Fax: (360) 236-4738

http://www.doh.wa.gov/nursing/

West Virginia—RN
West Virginia Board of Examiners
   for Registered Professional
   Nurses
101 Dee Drive
Charleston, West Virginia 25311
Phone: (304) 558-3596
Fax: (304) 558-3666

http://www.state.wv.us/nurses/rn/

Wisconsin
Wisconsin Department of
   Regulation & Licensing
1400 East Washington Avenue
P.O. Box 8935
Madison, Wisconsin 53708
Phone: (608) 266-0145
Fax: (608) 261-7083

http://www.state.wi.us/agencies/drl/

Wyoming
Wyoming State Board of Nursing
2020 Carey Avenue, Suite 110
Cheyenne, Wyoming 82002
Phone: (307) 777-7601
Fax: (307) 777-3519

http://nursing.state.wy.us/

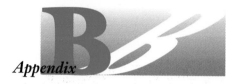

Specialty Nursing Organizations

Academy of Medical-Surgical Nurses
E. Holly Ave., Box 56
Pitman, NJ 08071-0056
856-256-2323
Fax: 856-589-7463
E-mail: amsn@ajj.com
Website: http://amsn.inurse.com

American Academy of Ambulatory Care Nursing
E. Holly Ave., Box 56
Pitman, NJ 08071-0056
1-800-262-6877
Fax: 586-589-7463
E-mail: aaacn@ajj.com
Website: http://aaacn.inurse.com

American Academy of Nurse Practitioners
P.O. Box 12846
Austin, TX 78711
512-442-4262
Fax: 512-442-6469
E-mail: admin@aanp.org
Website: http://www.aanp.org

American Academy of Nursing
600 Maryland Ave., SW
Suite 100 West
Washington, DC 20024-2571
202-651-7238
Fax: 202-554-2641
E-mail: tgaffney@ana.org
Website: http://www.nursingworld.org/aan

American Assembly for Men in Nursing
c/o NYSNA, 11 Cornell Rd.
Latham, NY 12110-1499
518-782-9400, ext. 346
E-mail: aamn@aamn.org
Website: http://www.aamn.org

American Association for the History of Nursing
P.O. Box 175
Lanoka Harbor, NJ 08734
609-693-7250
Fax: 609-693-1037
E-mail: aahn@aahn.org
Website: http://www.aahn.org

American Association of Colleges of Nursing
1 Dupont Circle, NW, Suite 530
Washington, DC 20036
202-463-6930
Fax: 202-785-8320
E-mail: webmaster@aacn.nche.edu
Website: http://www.aacn.nche.edu

American Association of Critical Care Nurses
101 Columbia
Aliso Viejo, CA 92656-1461
1-800-899-2226
Fax: 949-362-2020
E-mail: info@aacn.org
Website: http://www.aacn.org

American Association of Diabetes Educators
100 W. Monroe St., 4th Floor
Chicago, IL 60603-1901
312-424-2426
Fax: 312-424-2427
E-mail: aade@aadenet.org
Website: http://www.aadenet.org

American Association of Legal Nurse Consultants
4700 W. Lake Ave.
Glenview, IL 60025
877-402-2562
Fax: 847-375-6313
E-mail: info@aalnc.org
Website: http://www.aalnc.org

American Association of Neuroscience Nurses
4700 W. Lake Ave.
Glenview, IL 60025-1485
847-375-4733
Fax: 847-375-6333
E-mail: aann@aann.org
Website: http://www.aann.org

American Association of Nurse Anesthetists
222 S. Prospect Ave.
Park Ridge, IL 60068-4001
847-692-7050
Fax: 847-692-6968
E-mail: info@aana.com
Website: http://www.aana.com

The American Association of Nurse Attorneys
7794 Grow Dr.
Pensacola, FL 32514
850-474-3646
Fax: 850-484-8762
Website: http://www.taana.org

American Association of Occupational Health Nurses, Inc.
2920 Brandywine Rd., Suite 100
Atlanta, GA 30341
770-455-7757
Fax: 770-455-7271
E-mail: aaohn@aaohn.org
Website: http://www.aaohn.org

American Association of Office Nurses
109 Kinderkamack Rd.
Montvale, NJ 07645
1-800-457-7504
Fax: 201-573-8543
E-mail: aaonmail@aaon.org
Website: http://www.aaon.org

American Association of Spinal Cord Nurses
7520 Astoria Blvd.
Jackson Heights, NY 11370
718-803-3782
Fax: 718-803-0414
E-mail: info@epva.org
Website: http://www.aascin.org

American College of Nurse Practitioners
503 Capitol Court, NE, #300
Washington, DC 20002
202-546-4825
Fax: 202-546-4797
E-mail: acnp@nurse.org
Website: http://www.nurse.org/acnp

American Nephrology Nurses' Association
E. Holly Ave., Box 56
Pitman, NJ 08071-0056
1-888-600-2662
Fax: 856-589-7463
E-mail: anna@ajj.com
Website: http://anna.inurse.com

American Nurses Association
600 Maryland Ave. SW, Suite 100 West
Washington, DC 20024
1-800-274-4262
Fax: 202-651-7001
Website: http:// www.nursingworld.org

American Organization of Nurse Executives
1 N. Franklin
Chicago, IL 60606
312-422-2800
Fax: 312-422-4503
E-mail: aone@aha.org
Website: http://www.aone.org

American Psychiatric Nurses Association
1200 19th St., NW, Suite 300
Washington, DC 20036-2401
202-857-1133
Fax: 202-857-1102
E-mail: info@apna.org
Website: http://www.apna.org

American Society for Long-Term Care Nurses
660 Lonely Cottage Dr.
Upper Black Eddy, PA 18972-9313
610-847-5396
Fax: 610-847-5063

American Society of Pain Management Nurses
7794 Grow Dr.
Pensacola, FL 32514
1-888-342-7766
Fax: 850-484-8762
E-mail: aspmn@puetzamc.com
Website: http://www.aspmn.org

American Society of Perianesthesia Nurses
6900 Grove Rd.
Thorofare, NJ 08086
856-845-5557
Fax: 856-848-1881
E-mail: aspan@slackinc.com
Website: http://www.aspan.org

Association of Nurses in AIDS Care
11250 Roger Bacon Dr., Suite 8
Reston, VA 20190-5202
1-800-260-6780
Fax: 703-435-4390
E-mail: aidsnurses@aol.com
Website: http://www.anacnet.org

Association of Pediatric Oncology Nurses
4700 W. Lake Ave.
Glenview, IL 60025
847-375-4724
Fax: 847-375-6324
E-mail: info@apon.org
Website: http://www.apon.org

Association of Rehabilitation Nurses
4700 W. Lake Ave.
Glenview, IL 60025-1485
1-800-229-7530
Fax: 847-375-4777

Association of Women's Health, Obstetric, and Neonatal Nurses
2000 L St., NW, Suite 740
Washington, DC 20036
1-800-673-8499
Fax: 202-728-0575
Website: http://www.awhonn.org

Emergency Nurses Association
915 Lee St.
Des Plaines, IL 60016-6569
1-800-900-9659
Fax: 847-460-4001
E-mail: enainfo@ena.org
Website: http://www.ena.org

Endocrine Nurses Society
4350 E. West Hwy., Suite 500
Bethesda, MD 20814-4410
301-941-0249
Fax: 301-941-0259
E-mail: staff@endo-nurses.org
Website: http://www.endo-nurses.org

Home Healthcare Nurses Association
228 Seventh St., SE
Washington, DC 20003
1-800-558-4462
Fax: 202-547-3540
E-mail: hhna__info@nahc.org
Website: http://www.nahc.org/hhna

Hospice and Palliative Nurses Association
Medical Center East, Suite 375
211 N. Whitfield St.
Pittsburgh, PA 15206-3031
412-361-2470
Fax: 412-361-2425
Website: http://www.hpna.org

Intravenous Nurses Society
Fresh Pond Sq., 10 Fawcett St.
Cambridge, MA 02138
617-441-3008
Fax: 617-441-3009
Website: http://www.ins1.org

National Association of Clinical Nurse Specialists
4700 W. Lake Ave.
Glenview, IL 60025
847-375-4740
Fax: 847-375-4777
E-mail: info@nacns.org
Website: http://www.nacns.org

National Association of Hispanic Nurses
1501 16th St., NW
Washington, DC 20036
202-387-2477
Fax: 202-483-7183
E-mail: info@nahnhq.org
Website: http://nahnhq.org

National Association of Neonatal Nurses
701 Lee St., Suite 450
Des Plaines, IL 60016
1-800-451-3795
Fax: 847-297-6768
E-mail: info@nann.org
Website: http://www.nann.org

National Association of Orthopaedic Nurses
E. Holly Ave., Box 56
Pitman, NJ 08071-0056
856-256-2310
Fax: 856-589-7463
E-mail: naon@mail.ajj.com
Website: http://naon.inurse.com

National Association of School Nurses
P.O. Box 1300
Scarborough, ME 04070-1300
207-8832117
Fax: 207-883-2683
E-mail: nasn@nasn.org
Website: http://www.nasn.org

National Black Nurses Association, Inc.
8630 Fenton St., Suite 330
Silver Spring, MD 20910-3803
301-589-3200
Fax: 301-589-3223
E-mail: NBNA@erols.com
Website: http://www.nbna.org

National Council of State Boards of Nursing, Inc.
676 N. St. Clair St., Suite 550
Chicago, IL 60611-2921
312-787-6555
E-mail: info@ncsbn.org
Website: http://www.ncsbn.org

National Gerontological Nursing Association
7794 Grow Dr.
Pensacola, FL 32514
850-473-1174
Fax: 850-484-8762
E-mail: ngna@puetzamc.com
Website: http://www.ngna.org

National League for Nursing
61 Broadway, 33rd Floor
New York, NY 10006
1-800-669-1656
Fax: 212-812-0393
E-mail: nlnweb@nln.org
Website: http://www.nln.org

National Nursing Society on Addictions
4101 Lake Boone Trail,
Suite 201
Raleigh, NC 27607
919-783-5871
Fax: 919-787-4916
E-mail: info@nnsa.org
Website: http://www.nnsa.org

National Nursing Staff Development Organization
7794 Grow Dr.
Pensacola, FL 32514
1-800-489-1995
Fax: 850-484-8762

National Student Nurses' Association
555 W. 57th St.
New York, NY 10019
212-581-2211
Fax: 212-581-2368
E-mail: nsna@nsna.org
Website: http://www.nsna.org

Respiratory Nursing Society
7794 Grow Dr.
Pensacola, FL 32514-7072
850-474-8869
Fax: 850-484-8762
E-mail: rns@puetzamc.com

Society of Gastroenterology Nurses and Associates, Inc.
401 N. Michigan Ave.
Chicago, IL 60611-4267
1-800-245-7462
Fax: 312-527-6658
E-mail: shna@sba.com
Website: http://www.sgna.org

Society of Urologic Nurses and Associates
E. Holly Ave., Box 56
Pitman, NJ 08071-0056
1-888-827-7862
Fax: 856-589-7463
E-mail: suna@ajj.com

Website: http://www.suna.org

Wound, Ostomy, and Continence Nurses Society
1550 S. Coast Hwy., #201
Laguna Beach, CA 92651
1-888-224-9626
Fax: 949-376-3456
E-mail: maria@wocn.org

Website: http://www.wocn.org

Glossary of Terms

Academic shock   A feeling of being overwhelmed by the amount and complexity of schoolwork; may be manifested by behavioral changes such as passivity, aggression, depression, and self-neglect.

Advance directives   A written statement reflecting a person's choice regarding how health decisions should be made in the event he/she is unable to do so for himself/herself at a later time.

Advanced Practice Nurses   Nurses who have received at least a master's degree in nursing and who typically practice in a specialized role requiring further certification, such as a nurse practitioner, nurse midwife, or nurse anesthetist.

Advocate   Someone who protects and supports a person's right to make his/her own decisions; nurses act as client advocates regarding health care choices.

Alexian Brothers   An early male nursing organization; members administered to bubonic plague victims in 1348 and exist today in dual spiritual/nursing roles.

American Association of Colleges of Nursing   An organization that provides accreditation to baccalaureate nursing programs.

American Nurses' Association   A professional nursing organization that provides guidelines for safe, effective nursing practice to the public; also functions as a political voice for nursing.

Andragogy   The art of teaching as applied specifically to adults.

ANA Code of Ethics   A set of guidelines for nursing practice that describe the expected values and behaviors of the profession.

Assault   A threat to make bodily contact with someone without his/her consent.

Authority   The right to act in situations in which one is held accountable.

Autonomy   A client's right to make his/her own decision without coercion from others.

Barton, Clara   An early nursing leader; known as the organizer of the modern-day American Red Cross.

Battery   Intentional touching of another person without his/her permission.

Beneficence   The desire to "do good" when caring for clients.

Breckenridge, Mary   An early nursing leader who developed a frontier nurses' organization in rural Kentucky; the organization continues to provide midwifery care to remote areas.

Brown Report   A landmark report written by Esther Lucille Brown in 1948; it recommended that basic schools of nursing be placed in universities and colleges and that minorities and men be recruited into nursing.

Care provider   One component of nursing practice, it involves client care activities such as health screening and promotion and nursing interventions aimed at restoration of health.

Case manager   A nursing role that involves managing and coordinating health care services in a time- and cost-effective manner.

Change   The process of implementing new ideas, methods, or services within a group or institution.

Change agent   One who plays a primary role in implementing change in a group or institution.

Client teaching   The process of teaching clients/families about health promotion and restoration activities.

Client teaching plan   An outline for client teaching that includes an assessment of learning needs, client goals, teaching strategies, and methods to evaluate learning.

Clinical pathway   A multidisciplinary plan of client care that outlines the optimal sequencing and timing of intervention for particular diagnoses, procedures, or symptoms.

Collaborative problem   A client problem or complication that involves collaboration and care from more than one health care discipline; for example, physicians, nurses, nutritionists, and physical therapists would collaborate to work together to plan care for a pressure ulcer in a diabetic client.

Collaborator   One who works cooperatively with others toward a common purpose or goal.

Communication   The process of imparting information, exchanging ideas, and expressing one's self in such a way as to be understood.

Concept   A mental image of something; an abstract representation of an idea.

Conceptual model   A picture or graphic representation of concepts and their relationships.

Confidentiality   The act of protecting and keeping private all communications between caregivers and clients; information should be shared only with those members of the health care team who are involved in planning and delivering client care.

Conflict   A disagreement or struggle between two or more individuals regarding differing views, desires, or opinions.

Continuous quality improvement   A process of ongoing review of client care activities that seeks to ensure the delivery of quality care in a timely, cost-effective manner.

Counselor   One component of nursing practice that involves listening to client concerns and providing suggestions to assist in problem solving.

Creative thinking   A form of thinking that seeks to find new, unique ways to approach problems or accomplish tasks.

Critical thinking   A form of thinking that emphasizes logical, reflective consideration of what to believe or do.

Decision making   A thinking skill that involves making a selection of actions to achieve a particular outcome.

Delegation   The assignment of selected nursing tasks to competent persons in selected situations; the assignor retains accountability for ensuring that the tasks are carried out properly.

Deontology   An ethical theory based on the premise that all life is worthy of respect; right and wrong are clearly defined and are based on one's duty to follow moral rules.

Distress   Stress that causes negative effects in a person's life, such as illness.

Dix, Dorothea   An early nursing leader who campaigned for reforms in mental institutions; she was appointed superintendent of the Female Nurses of the Army during the American Civil War.

Dock, Lavinia   An early nursing leader who fought for women's rights issues and the right to vote.

Educator   A component of nursing practice that involves teaching clients, families, and communities health prevention, promotion, and restoration activities.

Entrepreneur   A business-like component of nursing practice whereby nurses function independently or interdependently to provide services such as consultation and education to clients and consumers.

Environment   The setting in which nursing care activities take place; also known as the sum of all conditions, influences, and circumstances affecting the person; social, spiritual, and cultural factors are included.

Ethical dilemma   A situation in which two or more ethical principles are in conflict and to which there is no obvious clear answer; both alternatives may result in equally unsatisfactory outcomes.

Eustress   Stress that causes positive changes in a person's life; usually consists of low levels of stress that motivate an increase in performance, such as schoolwork.

False imprisonment   Unauthorized use of force to hold another person against his/her wishes, such as detaining a client who desires to leave a hospital.

Fidelity   The duty to be faithful to commitments, such as keeping a promise not to divulge confidential information to others.

Front line manager   A manager who supervises nursing and ancillary personnel while managing client care as well; functions directly on client care units, such as a shift charge nurse or nursing team leader.

Health   A dynamic state of being; may change from day to day; may be viewed as a continuum with high-level wellness at one end and death at the other; people move from one point to another as factors affect health.

Hotel Dieu   A famous hospital in Paris operated by the Beguine religious order in the time of the Crusades; members of the order also cared for the ill in their homes.

Incident report   A form used to report an unusual or unexpected occurrence involving a client, visitor, or staff member in a health care facility or organization; may also be used to document equipment malfunction; a risk management tool.

Informed consent   Permission given by a client/designee for a procedure after having been fully informed by the physician of risks, benefits, potential complications, cost, and alternatives.

Interpersonal stressors   Factors that contribute to stressful interactions with others, such as neglecting to complete work assignments due to using work time to study for a test.

Intrapersonal stressors   Self-imposed concerns that cause stress, such as worrying about grades.

Justice   An ethical principle that refers to the fair treatment of everyone; all clients should have the right to expect the same level of care.

Knowledge domains   Three categories into which all learning processes may be divided; cognitive (knowledge level), affective (attitudes), and psychomotor (skills).

Knights Hospitalers of St. John of Jerusalem   A male religious order whose members provided care to ill travelers during the time of the Crusades in the Holy Land.

Knights of Saint Lazarus   A male religious order (established about 1200 C.E.) whose members dedicated themselves to caring for people with leprosy and syphilis.

Leadership   The ability to influence others in a manner that will get the job done.

Leadership styles   Three leadership styles proposed by Kurt Lewin; autocratic (leader-directed), democratic (leader and workers share decisions), and laissez faire (worker-directed).

Learning barriers   Factors that may impede learning in clients/families, such as illness, pain, and sensory deficits.

Life-cycle theory   A leadership theory proposed by Hersey and Blanchard that suggests that leadership style may be determined by the level of maturity or immaturity of the workers.

Malpractice   Negligence in the performance of professional duties; includes both acts of commission and omission.

Managed care   A system of health care in which a specified group of people receive services for a predetermined fixed fee.

Management   Planning, organizing, directing, coordinating, and controlling activities designed to meet organizational goals.

Manager   A component of nursing practice that involves supervisory, planning, and coordinating activities for other nursing staff, groups of clients, families, and communities.

Mentor   A function of nursing practice in which a nurse guides, supports, and promotes professional growth in a less experienced nurse.

Metacognition   The process of analyzing one's own thought processes in order to ensure better thinking.

Middle manager   A manager, such as a unit nurse manager, who supervises personnel of the front line level and who is usually responsible for budgetary, staffing, and quality care issues.

Montag, Mildred   A nursing leader who promoted creation of the associate degree as a shorter route into nursing.

National Council of State Boards of Nursing   An organization responsible for developing test questions and setting minimum pass rates for nursing licensure.

National League for Nursing   A nursing organization formed in 1893, originally to provide standards of education for nursing programs; today, the organization also offers workshops and seminars, accredits nursing programs, and provides curriculum consultation.

National Student Nurses' Association   A professional organization for nursing students that was formed in 1952; representatives may serve on selected committees of the American Nurses' Association.

NCLEX-PN   The national licensing exam for graduates of practical/vocational nursing programs.

NCLEX-RN   The national licensing exam for graduates of registered nursing programs.

Networking   Sharing information and ideas with other members of the profession in order to build positive relationships with peers that foster better communication.

Nightingale, Florence   A nineteenth-century Englishwoman who is known as the founder of modern nursing; her contributions to nursing include educational standards and improvement in the status of nurses.

Nonmaleficence   An ethical principle that means to inflict no harm.

Nontraditional student   A student in a program of study who does not fall within the traditional demographic description of a college/university student (between 18 and 22 years of age, supported by parents, single, no children).

Nonverbal communication   Communication between individuals in ways other than verbal language, such as gestures, facial expressions, and body stance.

North American Nursing Diagnosis Association (NANDA)   A group that was formed in 1970 for the purpose of developing a comprehensive list of nursing diagnoses; the list is revised every few years.

Nurse Practice Act   A law defining the scope of practice within a given state.

Nursing   The diagnosis and treatment of human responses to actual or potential health problems; activities and interactions with clients aimed at promoting or restoring health, as well as assisting with a peaceful death.

Nursing diagnosis   A diagnostic statement that describes a client or community response to an actual or potential health problem; also includes wellness diagnoses.

Nursing Interventions Classification (NIC)   A comprehensive standardized language that describes the treatments that nurses perform.

Nursing Outcomes Classification (NOC)   A standardized classification system of client outcomes that are responsive to nursing care.

Nursing process   The use of nursing knowledge and skills to formulate a plan of care for a client or community; the process is problem-oriented and involves input from the client and family.

Nutting, Mary Adelaide   An early nursing leader, author of a nursing history, and first professor of nursing.

Objective data   Assessment data collected by using the five senses, also known as signs; is usually considered to be measurable.

Patient Self-Determination Act   A legislative act that went into effect in 1991; calls for health care organizations to make patients aware of their right to determine personal end-of-life options.

Pedagogy   The science and practice of teaching.

Person   The recipient of nursing care; may refer to an individual, family, group, or community.

Philosophy   The study of basic principles and truths.

Power   The ability to influence others to do something they would not normally do.

Problem solving   Working out a correct solution to a problem; resolving or answering a proposed question.

Professional socialization   The process of developing an identity within a chosen profession.

Proposition   A statement that describes a relationship between two or more concepts.

Researcher   A component of nursing practice that involves investigating possible solutions to nursing and/or client problems.

Richards, Linda   The first graduate of an American nursing school.

Risk management   The process of identifying, evaluating, and reducing actual or potential legal problems in a health care setting.

Robb, Isabel Hampton   A nursing leader who reduced working hours of students, promoted licensure exams, and helped establish early nursing organizations.

Role   A culturally learned pattern of behavior.

Role conflict   An emotional struggle experienced when one perceives incompatible role requirements.

Role model   An individual who demonstrates behavior that is desirable of a member of a given group or profession.

Role transition   Activities aimed at shaping, modifying, and adding information as a new role is assumed.

Statutory laws   Laws established through a formal legislative process; includes both criminal and civil laws.

Stress   A nonspecific response of the body to any demand made upon it; may be due to physical, emotional, spiritual, or other factors.

Subjective data   Assessment data that is verbally expressed by the client; also known as symptoms.

Survival skills   Activities and behaviors aimed at assisting students to achieve a healthy balance between school, work, and home life.

Teleology   An ethical theory based on the premise that what is useful is good; emphasis is placed on results, not moral principles of right and wrong.

Theory   A general explanation of why something occurs.

Therapeutic communication   A unique form of communication between a client and nurse that fosters mutual respect and self-worth.

Thinking skills   Mental activities that help nurses assist clients to achieve expected outcomes, such as critical thinking, creative thinking, problem solving, and decision making.

Time management   Effective organization of time so responsibilities are completed as desired.

Top-level manager   The administrative level of management, usually made up of the board of directors, chief executive officer, and vice presidents of the organization.

Traditional student   A student who fits the typical demographics of a college student: between 18 and 23 years of age, single, unemployed, and financially dependent on parents.

Transformational leadership   A leadership style that focuses on rewarding for quality and excellence, rather than on punishing and manipulating to achieve outcomes; the leader maintains a positive attitude that concentrates on success.

Values   Personal beliefs and attitudes regarding what is important.

Veracity   The duty to tell the truth.

Wald, Lillian   An early nursing leader who founded public health nursing.

Index

Note: Page numbers followed by f indicate figures; those followed by t indicate tables; and those followed by b indicate boxed material.